# IAN WRIGHT'S
# FITTER
# FAMILIES

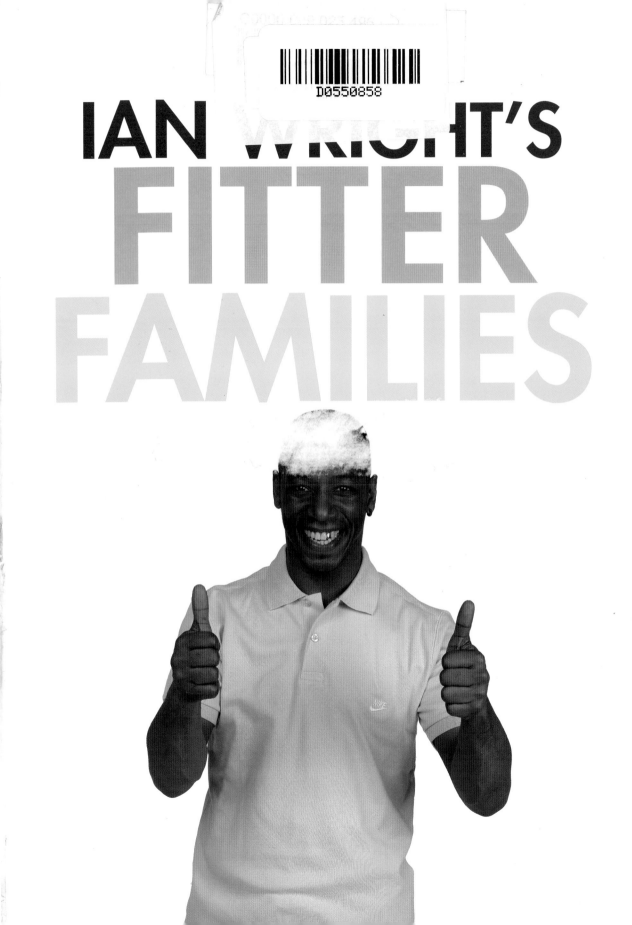

First published 2008 by
A & C Black Publishers Ltd
38 Soho Square, London W1D 3HB
www.acblack.com

Copyright © 2008 Ian Wright and Dean Horridge with
Anita Bean

ISBN 978-1-408-10696-9

A CIP catalogue record for this book is available from the
British Library.

Note: It is always the responsibility of the individual to
assess his or her own fitness capability before participating
in any training activity. Whilst every effort has been made
to ensure the content of this book is as techincally accurate
as possible, neither the author nor the publishers can
accept responsibility for any injury or loss sustained as a
result of the use of this material.

All the internet addresses given in this book were correct
at the time of going to press. The author and the publishers
regret any inconvenience caused if addresses have
changed or sites have ceased to exist, but can accept
no responsibility for any such changes.

Ian Wright is represented by the SEM Group,
98 Cockfosters Road, Barnet, Herts EN4 0DP
(020 8447 4250; www.semplc.com).

Created by Bookwork Ltd, Stroud, UK
Cover design by James Watson
New photography by Andy Crawford
Manufactured by South China Printing Company Ltd, China

This book is produced using paper that is made from
wood grown in managed, sustainable forests. It is natural,
renewable and recyclable. The logging and manufacturing
processes conform to the environmental regulations of the
country of origin.

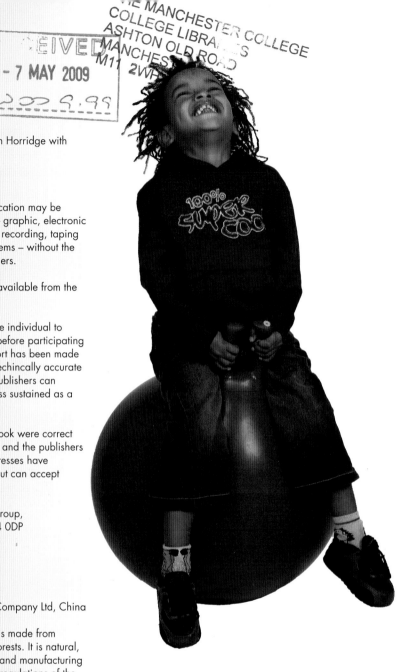

# "In 1971, 80% of 7- and 8-year-olds walked to school. By 1991, the figure was 9%."

# Contents

**5** CHAPTER 1
THE RIGHT TIME FOR CHANGE

6 This is the SAS approach
8 Small changes, big results
10 Leading the way for change
12 Making changes as a family
14 What does it mean to be fit?
16 So what's stopping you?
18 Set goals
20 Make a family commitment
22 Putting the plan into practice

**25** CHAPTER 2
HOW YOU CAN STAY ACTIVE

26 How much, how often?
28 A word before you start
30 Prepare for action
32 Choosing your activities
34 Exercise in your own time
38 Exercise while you work
41 Getting around
43 Exercising together
46 Indoor activities
48 Ian's family fun
52 More family fun
57 Even more ideas
58 Safety first
60 Reward yourself

**63** CHAPTER 3
EAT HEALTHILY TO STAY FIT

64 Small steps to good habits
66 What about my weight?
68 Six weeks to a healthier you
70 Eating the right way
76 Trim the fat

78 Cut down on the sugar
81 Eat less salt
82 What your body needs
86 Five a day
89 What's in your lunchbox today?
90 Healthy store cupboard
92 Start with breakfast
94 Lunch on the run
96 Dinner time made easy
99 Just a snack between meals
100 Takeaways and eating out
104 A little of what you fancy

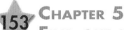

**107** CHAPTER 4
ACTION STATIONS!

108 On your feet
110 Build up gradually
113 Take a hike!
114 Made it!
116 Come along for the ride
118 Pace yourself
120 Hit the ground running
122 Running for fun
125 Sink or swim
126 In the swim
128 Fun for all the family
147 Balloon-tastic!
148 Home challenge for everyone
150 Keeping active at work too!

**153** CHAPTER 5
FIND OUT MORE

154 Useful websites
158 A final word
160 Acknowledgements

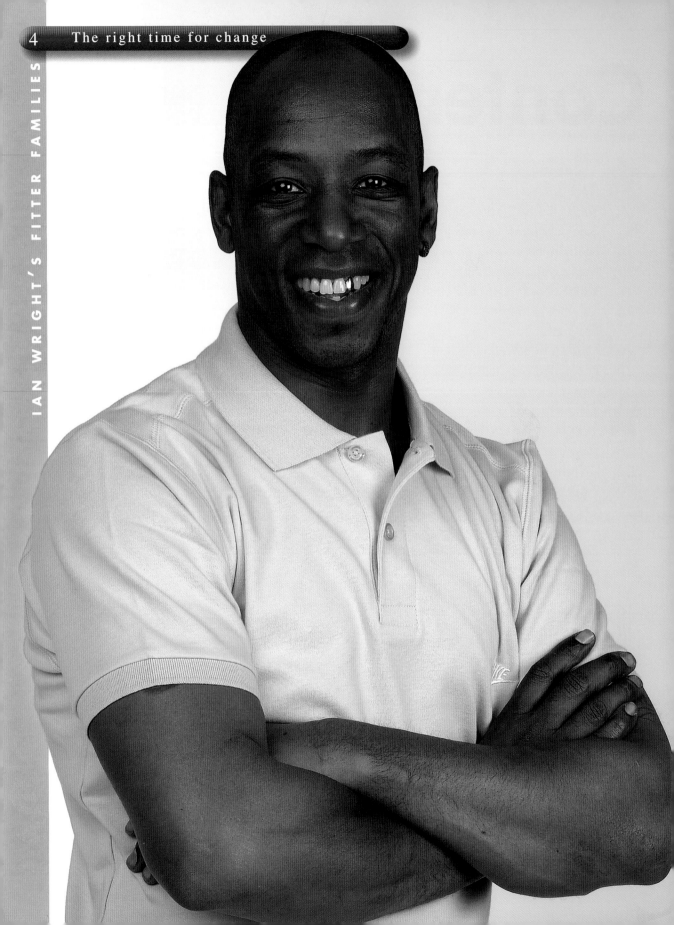

# The right time for change

We've got a major obesity, health and **fitness problem** in Britain. Unless we do something now, 60 per cent of us will be obese by 2050. That's why I wanted to write this book. We have to teach kids why **it's important** to be fit, and show them how. It's about being a good role model, getting off the couch and **getting fit together**.

**Myths & Facts**

**FACT:** The number of overweight kids in Britain has doubled in ten years. One in three primary school leavers is overweight.

IAN WRIGHT'S FITTER FAMILIES

# This is the SAS approach

I'm not asking you to run a marathon, or win a football match, or even jog around the park, if that's not your bag. Getting fit is all about making **simple** changes in your daily life, setting yourself achievable goals and knowing that you will be able to sustain them. That's the SAS approach. **Simple**, **Achievable**, **Sustainable**. Easy.

## SAS
### SIMPLE
### ACHIEVABLE
### SUSTAINABLE

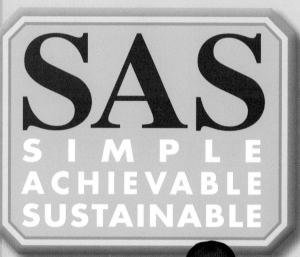

**Wherever you see the symbol above ...** *it will remind you what fitness is all about. SAS applies to every change you make, whether it's taking a little exercise each day or eating more healthily.*

The idea behind this book is that the goals you set as a family should be SAS. Don't try to bite off more than you can chew. Exercise can and should be fun.

### SIMPLE
Keep every goal simple. Don't set yourself goals that are too big or complicated, because you will never achieve them.

### ACHIEVABLE
If your goal is too hard, you'll make excuses and then give up. On the other hand, if it's too easy, you won't set yourself another goal.

### SUSTAINABLE
Any change you make has to fit into your lifestyle long-term. Make sure you can keep up those healthy habits every day and every week.

⭐ Aim to achieve one thing at a time. Taking a 50-metre walk every day is a great start. Keep that up, then take on another challenge.

⭐ Exercise can and should be fun. Pick activities that you enjoy – that way you'll keep them up.

⭐ Encourage kids to have a go and have fun. If they enjoy exercise they are more likely to continue a healthy lifestyle as an adult.

### OBESITY

Nearly a quarter of British adults are now obese. Being obese means being so overweight that your health is in danger. You risk dying young, developing heart disease, cancer or diabetes. The problem has rocketed three-fold since 1980, and there's no sign that the upward trend is slowing. Children are also getting fatter, which means they're storing up a lot of health problems. They're more likely to suffer high blood pressure and Type-2 diabetes in their teens. And they're more likely to be teased, bullied and suffer low self-esteem.

**All the family**
*When everyone joins in and pulls together, it's easier to keep going. It's also more fun exercising together and trying to outdo each other!*

**TOP TIP**
Even if you are already active, you can still benefit by adding more activity. The more active you are, the more benefits you will get!

# Small changes, big results

I'm not saying it's easy to change old habits. But if you set yourself **SAS** goals **you can do it**. Take small steps at first – every change you make, no matter how small, counts. In the end the small changes will all add up to make **big, positive changes**.

**E**very day, ask yourself – what can I do today to eat more healthily and move more? Look for small ways to meet your goals every day, because every little step counts towards a better, fitter future.

### EASY DOES IT!

Start small and go slowly. Small changes are a lot easier to stick with than drastic ones. Walking one mile or cutting out one biscuit could save you 100 calories. If you do that every day for a year, it adds up to enough calories to prevent the annual 1kg weight gain that happens to most adults.

### BE A FITTER FAMILY

Get the whole family involved. If you can all make that commitment to fitness, you'll see the results more quickly. Start doing simple activities, such as walking, cycling and swimming together. Whether it's walking to school, walking the dog together, going on a family bike ride or kicking a ball around in the garden, you'll be working as a team. You can support one another and urge each other on. A little bit of family competition is healthy and will help you to meet your goals. Making changes together means you're more likely to keep them up. And it's heaps more fun that way!

*Myths*

**FACT**: Half an hour playing Frisbee increases your heart rate and burns about 100 calories – equivalent to four squares of chocolate.

*Facts*

#### Little by little
*When you pour a glass of water into a bath it doesn't look like it's making any difference to how much water's in there. But if you keep pouring glasses of water in, it all adds up and the bath starts to fill up. The same is true for exercise and your fitness.*

# Leading the way for change

Lead by example. If you **show your kids** that you are active then they will want to be active as well. You are a role model for your children. **They should see that you exercise** and eat a healthy diet. Better still, do activities together!

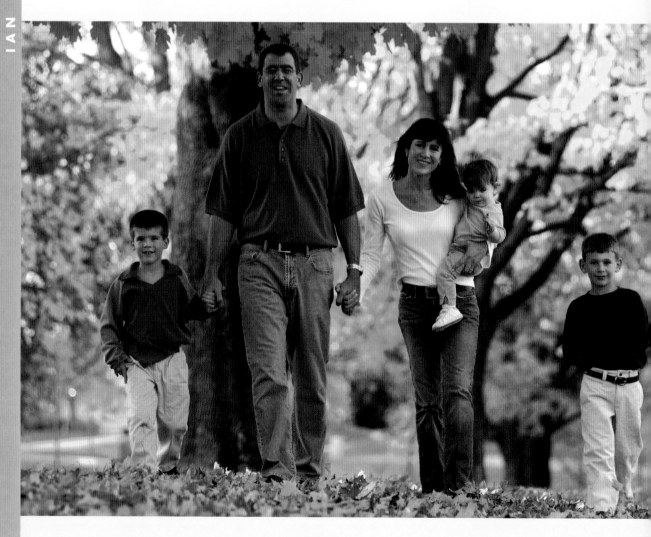

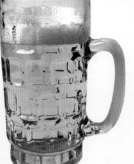

**Treats**
*The odd pint of beer or a cheeky ice cream isn't the end of the world.*

**Fit day out**
*A family walk is an excellent way of exploring the great outdoors and getting fit too.*

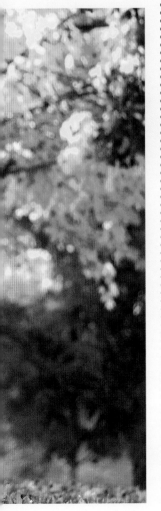

**Y**our kids' days should be as action-packed as possible. Walking to and from school and other nearby places, riding a bike to visit friends and playing active games will help them see exercise as a way of life. Keep it fun – it's important that kids have fun with activities they do. If they're enthusiastic about activities and sport then they'll stick to them.

### SET REALISTIC GOALS

Ensure that the goals you set are realistic and achievable. It might sound obvious but if you ask yourself or your kids to do something that's too hard, then you'll be disappointed. Don't quit just because an activity is new or because you've eaten something that's not very healthy. You can still have the occasional chocolate bar or glass of wine. Don't tell yourself you can never have these things or you won't stick to it. The important thing is that you don't go overboard.

# "It doesn't have to be hell to be healthy."

### START WITH WALKING

Instead of trying to achieve the government's 'out of school' guideline of two to three hours of exercise per week immediately, set steady goals that build up over a few months to three hours per week. This way the exercise will become part of a routine and the gradual change will barely be noticed. Children will feel better and be able to do more. Start with walking to school as much as possible or getting off the bus earlier.

### JUST GET ACTIVE

If sport is not your child's thing, try out aerobic classes, swimming, dance or martial arts. It's not just sport that can make a difference. Walking, cycling and even gardening are all forms of activity that can help your family to lead a more active lifestyle. Be positive – there is something out there for everyone.

### LACK OF EXERCISE

Seven out of ten children are driven to school even though they live less than a mile away, according to a 2006 survey of 5- to 12-year-old children. Less than 1% of children cycle to school, and more than 80% watch more than one hour of television each day during the school week.

# Making changes as a family

Committing together and making small healthy **lifestyle changes** will result in you becoming a fitter family. Kids learn eating and exercise habits from their parents. They are more likely to copy **what you do** than what you say.

## Myths & Facts

**FACT:** Children of active parents are more likely to become active themselves. You will help them as well as yourself if you are a role model.

**D**on't worry if you can't run a mile or swim ten lengths or even dance the tango! The important thing is that you're not afraid to have a go. Always try your best – that's good enough.

### THIS IS YOUR CHANCE FOR CHANGE

This is your family's chance for change. Show your kids that you are all in it together by making small changes to the whole family's eating and activity habits. Over time, these new routines will become part of day-to-day life. Everyone will feel better, become fitter and may lose weight.

### MAKE EXERCISE FUN FOR THE WHOLE FAMILY

Encourage your kids to pick activities they enjoy. Provide lots of simple play kit at home – balls, skipping ropes, Frisbees and bikes. Introduce them to as many different activities and sports as you can – football, racquet games, swimming, dance lessons …

- You and your family are embarking on a long-term effort to become more active and feel fitter.
- You will succeed by taking small steps and giving each other lots of encouragement.
- This is a serious commitment, but that doesn't mean it's boring – have fun while taking part in activities and exercise.

### REMEMBER: SAS!

Your target setting must include the Simple, Achievable and Sustainable method throughout. Each family member may have a different fitness or activity level, which must be taken into consideration when forming the Family Weekly Plan (see page 22).

Opposite: Walking the dog
*Get outside and get some fresh air and exercise by walking the dog. Or borrow a friend's dog!*

### OVERWEIGHT CHILDREN

One in three children under 10 is overweight or obese. Contrary to popular belief, most of them don't shed their puppy fat. Six in ten chubby pre-schoolers will be overweight by the time they are 12. And overweight teenagers have a 70% chance of becoming an overweight adult.

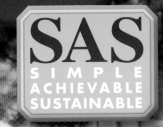

**SAS**

SIMPLE
ACHIEVABLE
SUSTAINABLE

# What does it mean to be fit?

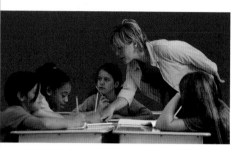

**Fit makes you smarter!**
*Being fitter boosts your brain power. It means you'll be able to concentrate better at work. Kids will do better in school and may even finish their homework more easily.*

Getting fit is **not about hard work** or punishing yourself. You don't have to give up eating all the things you love to be fit, and you **don't have to be thin**. Look at professional rugby players. They are super fit, but they are **certainly not thin**!

## HOW WILL YOU FEEL WHEN YOU'RE FIT?

Being fit gives you more confidence in yourself. When you are fit you not only look good but feel great too.

- You'll feel less tired and have lots more energy.
- Being fit helps kids to concentrate, which means they will do better in school.
- Your body is more able to fight off germs that make you ill.

## WHY DO YOU NEED TO BE FIT?

There are loads of great reasons for getting more active. Here are just some of them.

- To feel good about yourself
- To strengthen your heart and lungs
- To get stronger muscles
- To feel less tired and have lots more energy
- To live longer and cut your risk of certain diseases, such as heart disease
- To strengthen your bones and reduce the risk of osteoporosis
- To give you more confidence
- To feel happier and help you cope better under stress

## BEING FIT MEANS ...

⭐ You **can** still eat a bacon sandwich, but swap to wholemeal bread and add in some fresh tomato and salad.

⭐ You **can** still have ice cream, but just not every day!

## IT DOESN'T MEAN ...

⭐ You don't have to go to the gym. Exercise should be enjoyable not a punishment. Work within your limits, start slowly and build over time.

⭐ You don't have to spend a fortune. Just adding more activity to your daily life gets you fit — for free.

⭐ You don't have to give up the things you enjoy. Start with small changes – you can still have a little chocolate.

### TOO LITTLE ACTIVITY
Only three out of ten boys and four out of ten girls are meeting the recommended one hour of daily activity.

Not a good sarnie!
*Remember, wholemeal bread and a bit of salad would make this bacon sarnie much more healthy!*

# So what's stopping you?

Making the effort to build more activity into your life might seem like hard work. It's easy to make excuses, but **you will get fitter** only when you **open your mind** to the possibility that **you can** get fitter. If you believe you can, you will. If you believe you can't, you probably won't.

Y ou will have plenty of excuses for putting off until tomorrow your plans to lose weight and get fitter. But with the health time-bomb ticking, you need to start making changes today. Throw out your excuses and start thinking more positively. Here are some simple ways to change your mindset.

### I DON'T HAVE TIME

Make time to get fit! It needn't be time-consuming. Build activity into your daily routine. Walk to work or school, use the stairs instead of the lift, cycle to the shops – it all adds up.

### I HAVEN'T GOT ENOUGH WILLPOWER

Set Simple, Achievable and Sustainable goals and you'll have the willpower. Only if your goals are too demanding will your willpower fade.

### EXERCISE IS TOO HARD

It won't feel hard if you choose the right activities and work at a comfortable pace. No one's telling you to sprint up a hill. Start slowly and build up.

### MY FAMILY ARE FAT SO I WILL BE TOO

If you do nothing, then you probably will be fat too. But if you start eating healthily and exercise regularly you can overcome family trends.

### I'VE GOT A SLOW METABOLISM

It's been proven that fat people have a higher metabolism than thin people. To lose weight you have to take in fewer calories than you burn.

### IT COSTS TOO MUCH MONEY

You don't need an expensive gym membership. There are loads of free things you can start to do to get yourself fitter.

IAN WRIGHT'S FITTER FAMILIES

**SO WHAT ARE YOU WAITING FOR? COME ON, NO MORE EXCUSES!**

The reason why some people succeed and others don't is less to do with talent or luck and more to do with how they think. In competitive sport, for example, the difference between the winners and the losers can be very small. It's their mindset that makes the difference.

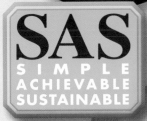

**SAS**
**SIMPLE ACHIEVABLE SUSTAINABLE**

# Set goals

Have you ever **tried to lose weight**, do a sponsored run or challenge yourself to reach **some other goal**? Maybe everything went really well to start with, but then you lost some of that drive and had **trouble getting motivated** again.

**E**veryone struggles to stay motivated and reach their goals. Just look at how many people go on diets, lose weight and then pile it back on again! The truth is that making any change is a big deal. But it's not impossible. With the right approach, you can definitely do it.

## WHY IT'S IMPORTANT TO SET GOALS

Setting goals is important. Without them you are in danger of being full of good intentions but without a practical plan of action. Research has shown that people who set good goals are more likely to be successful in making changes.

## HOW TO SET GOALS

To be successful, your goals have to be Simple, Achievable and Sustainable. SAS! They have to fit into your life. If they're too hard you won't reach them. It's important to break big goals (say, to run 5km) into smaller goals (say, to run 500 metres, then 1km and so on). Go at your own steady pace. Each time you reach a small goal, you set yourself another small goal until you reach your big goal. That's how you build up your fitness.

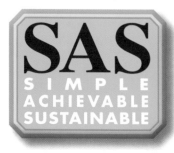

**SAS**
SIMPLE
ACHIEVABLE
SUSTAINABLE

## GOAL SETTING MADE EASY

Setting goals isn't rocket science but it does take a bit of thought. The first step is to assess where you are now and where you want to be. Then write it down in as much detail as possible. A good goal is made of five elements:

**Specific** It's easier to plan for and achieve a specific goal than a vague one.

**Measurable** You need to measure your progress otherwise you won't know whether you have reached your goal.

**Agreed** Commit your goal to paper. You will be more likely to achieve it than if you simply keep it as a thought.

**Realistic** There's nothing wrong with aiming for the top, but be realistic.

**Time-scaled** Set a clear and realistic timescale with specific daily tasks.

## MAKE A CONTRACT WITH FITNESS

Put your goal in writing. Writing down a goal is part of the mental process of committing to it. You should also write down the reasons why you want to achieve that goal and how achieving it will improve your life. Look at your goal every day to keep you focused and to remind you how much you want to achieve it.

**MY GOAL IS** ....................................................................
................................................................................
................................................................................
................................................................................

**I WANT TO ACHIEVE MY GOAL BECAUSE** ...............
................................................................................
................................................................................
................................................................................
................................................................................
................................................................................
................................................................................
................................................................................

# Make a family commitment

To be a **fitter family**, you all need to agree to make changes to your routine. By signing a **commitment to fitness**, you are more likely to stay motivated and be able to achieve your **goals**.

The whole family should sign this commitment to fitness although the terms are for different people. Terms 1 and 2 are for children, terms 3 to 7 are for parents or guardians and terms 8 to 10 are for the whole family.

**1** You will try to do some form of daily exercise and update the weekly planner honestly once it has been completed.

**2** You will commit to making the right food choices and will encourage others in the family to do the same.

**3** You will motivate and support your family and work towards the SAS approach, remembering you are a role model.

**4** You will show to the family your own dedication and commitment to the programme and the benefits it offers you and your family.

**5** You will apply the healthy lifestyle factors that your family have agreed to at home, work or play, so they are as consistent as possible.

**6** You will help your family to make the right food choices, starting with your weekly trip to the supermarket.

**7** You will encourage your children to be more active at home and school, with limits on TV and computer games.

**8** You will aim to have a healthier, more active lifestyle, both in terms of what you eat and the exercise you do.

**9** You will make an effort to meet your goals and stay fully committed to meeting them on a long-term basis.

**10** You will always try your best. When the going gets tough you will persevere instead of giving up.

Each member of the family should agree and sign below.

Signed ............................................. Dated ....../......./.......
Signed ............................................. Dated ....../......./.......
Signed ............................................. Dated ....../......./.......
Signed ............................................. Dated ....../......./.......
Signed ............................................. Dated ....../......./.......

This agreement should be revisited and discussed in times of dispute. In addition, if goals are not being achieved by any member of the family, the necessary changes can be agreed.

IAN WRIGHT'S FITTER FAMILIES

## Myths & Facts

**FACT:** In the UK, less than 3% of children exercise regularly. Only 1 in 250 girls and 1 in 20 boys are active enough to stay healthy.

**WHERE THERE'S SMOKE ...**
Active kids are also less likely to become smokers – another reason to get fitter.

# Putting the plan into practice

Try to meet as a family once a week. The weekend is a **good time** to **discuss and plan**. Everyone in the family should be given a chance to have their say and set their own goals. Get everyone to list their favourite activities and perhaps suggest some **new ones** they'd like to try.

**K**eep focusing on the SAS approach. Try to avoid expensive activities and keep it simple. Place your family plan somewhere prominent, such as on the fridge, so everyone can see it and check off their activities. Here are some ideas to get you started on making your plan.

| FAMILY MEMBER | DAY ONE | DAY TWO | DAY THREE | DAY FOUR | DAY FIVE | DAY SIX | DAY SEVEN |
|---|---|---|---|---|---|---|---|
| MUM | Walk to work | | Get off the bus one stop earlier and walk | | Eat a healthy lunch | Walk the dog | |
| DAD | Use the stairs, not the lift | Eat a piece of fruit | | Walk the dog | | | Cycle to the shops |
| THOMAS | PE lesson | | Walk the dog | Don't have any fizzy drinks | | Play football with mates | |
| LIZZIE | Walk the dog | | PE lesson | Eat a piece of fruit | | Watch only one hour of TV | |
| FITTER FAMILY TIME | Healthy family dinner | | Healthy family dinner | | Walk to the local park | | Walk the dog together |

## HOW TO PROGRESS YOUR GOALS

Even if you all do just one activity a week, that's a good start. The following week, you should add another activity or aim to do the first activity for longer.

## FAMILY WEEKLY MEETING

At your family meeting, discuss the week's achievements. Did you do all the things you set out to do? Were they too hard or too easy? How did you feel? Then plan what you will do the following week.

★ Show the achievements on the Weekly Family Plan.

★ Get everyone to reflect on the previous week. What went well and maybe not so well?

★ Help each other to set goals for next week, but don't try to run a marathon when you should be walking a mile.

★ Keep the meetings short and sweet. Remember, this is time when you could be active.

★ Always praise even when targets are not achieved. Trying your best is always good enough.

★ If anyone has failed to achieve their weekly goals, don't give them a hard time. Encourage them to make a better effort next week.

★ If anyone keeps on falling short of their goals, yet tries their best, then they are probably setting their goals too high and need to set new SAS ones.

**Achievable goals**
*As one of your goals, aim to have a piece of fruit instead of a fizzy drink. It all adds up!*

IAN WRIGHT'S FITTER FAMILIES

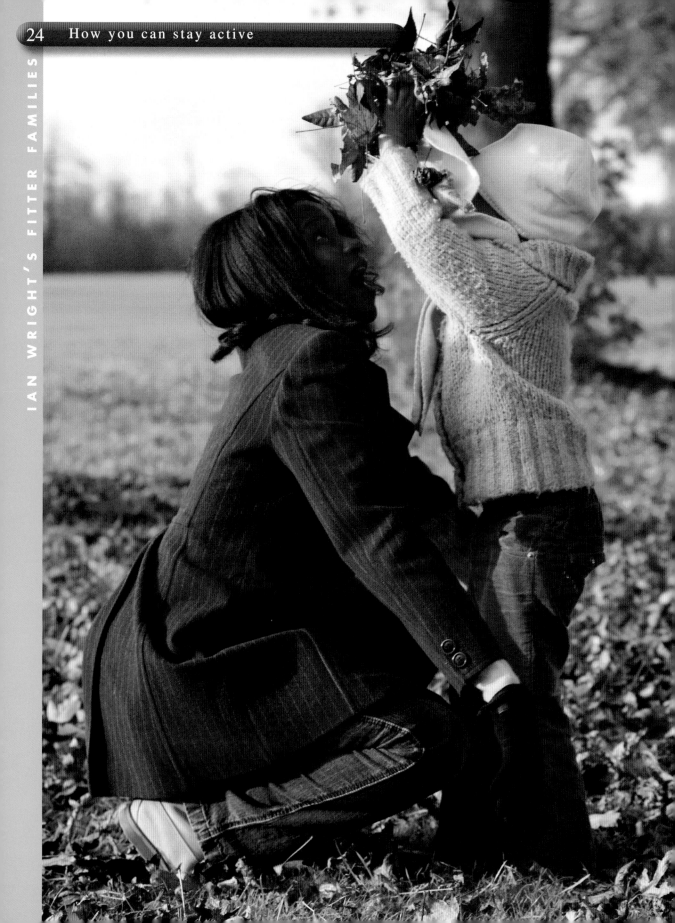

# How you can stay active

Getting more active **as a family** gets you fit and also improves your relationship with your kids and partner. It's **more motivating and more fun** when you exercise together. You can encourage each other, compete with each other and celebrate your achievements together. Exercising as a family is **more sustainable** than going it alone.

*Myths*

**FACT:** It is important to increase your physical activity gradually – both the amount of time you spend doing it, and the intensity.

*Facts*

# How much, how often?

Try to **move your body** at every opportunity. It doesn't matter for how long. The main thing is that you gradually **build a little** more activity into your day.

## "Three 10-minute sessions of exercise produce the same results as one 30-minute one."

Choose an activity and do it as often as you can and for as long as feels comfortable. Then build it up gradually – an extra walk here, an extra swim with the kids there. It'll challenge your body and you'll soon get fitter.

### How much exercise?

Aim to do something active every day. Experts recommend adults spending 30 minutes and kids spending an hour doing some kind of activity that makes you breathe faster and your heart beat faster on at least five days a week. But start off with just ten minutes if that's all you can manage. Then build up gradually to your 30-minute target.

### Getting started

Take it easy to begin with. Exercise should never feel painful or leave you completely puffed out. If you push yourself too hard you risk injuring yourself and you will want to give up.

- If you can have a leisurely conversation while you exercise, you probably aren't working hard enough.
- If you can barely gasp a word, slow down!
- Begin slowly for the first few minutes and build up gradually – this will help protect your muscles and joints from injury.
- Cool down gradually when you come to the end of your activity.

## MOVING
### FOR FITNESS

It's important for kids to move about for at least one hour every day. They don't have to do this all in one go – they can split up the hour through the day. Activities could include walking to and from school, playing with their friends, playing sport or any of the fun activities in this book. If they are put off by the thought of exercise, make the activities seem part of everyday life rather than a task.

**SAS**
SIMPLE
ACHIEVABLE
SUSTAINABLE

### Work your way up
*Don't overdo it and suddenly start roller-blading every day. You won't be able to sustain it.*

### Start young
*Activity is essential for kids from a very young age to help them develop healthily.*

# A word before you start

**TOP TIP**

You don't need expensive clothing for taking exercise, but be comfortable. Your trainers should feel roomy around the toes, be flexible, provide cushioning around the heel and feel comfortable and light. In warm weather, wear light, loose clothing such as a T-shirt and shorts or tracksuit bottoms. In cold weather, wear layers so that you can remove the outer ones as you get warm – a fleece or sweatshirt over a T-shirt.

Just thinking about getting more active is **an important first step**. Don't let negative thoughts or other people's views put you off getting started. **It might be difficult** to ignore them but remember, getting fit is all about improving **your** health. Take that step for your sake and **your family's sake**.

## Myths & Facts

**MYTH:** No pain, no gain. Not true! Pain is your body's way of telling you something is wrong. Pain means it's time to slow down or stop.

Before you get moving, make sure you've got the basics covered. You don't need flashy kit or an expensive gym membership. For most activities all you need is a pair of comfortable trainers (or flat shoes if you're walking) and suitable clothing. For everything else, keep it as simple as possible.

### A WORD BEFORE YOU START

Consult your doctor if you have a health problem, such as heart disease, asthma, arthritis or diabetes. Also talk to the doctor if you have back problems or if you're not used to taking exercise. He or she will advise you about your level of physical activity.

**Stay in bed**
*If you're under the weather it's not always a good idea to get up and exercise.*

### WHEN NOT TO EXERCISE

There are times when you shouldn't exercise. Listen to your body's warning signs if you are feeling ill or hungry or in discomfort.

- Don't push yourself if you are unwell. It's a myth that you can 'sweat out' a cold.
- Don't exercise if you've got, or are recovering from, a viral illness like flu, if you need to take pain killers or if you have a medical condition and haven't talked to your doctor first.
- Stop exercising if you have difficulty breathing, get any pain in your chest, neck and/or upper left arm.
- Stop exercising if you feel dizzy, sick or unwell, or very tired.
- Don't exercise on an empty stomach.
- Wait about two hours after eating before taking any exercise.

### TEST YOUR FITNESS

Many health and fitness websites have useful tools like calorie counters, body-mass index tables and pre-exercise fitness tests. Log on to www.netfit.co.uk for fitness programmes.

IAN WRIGHT'S FITTER FAMILIES

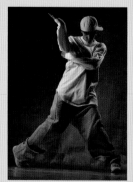

**Dance 'til you drop**
*Dancing to your favourite music is a great way to work out – and, even if you're not the world's greatest dancer, it's guaranteed to put a grin on your face!*

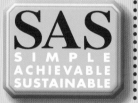

**SAS**
SIMPLE
ACHIEVABLE
SUSTAINABLE

# Prepare for action

**Most of us** can find time to watch a film, go out for a drink or play games on the computer. But for many people, **finding time** to exercise is more difficult! It helps when the exercise is **enjoyable**.

### GET READY FOR ACTION
If the thought of putting on your trainers leaves you cold, these 'go get it' tips will help you.

- Do it with someone else – your kids, your partner or a buddy – exercising with someone else is more fun than going it alone.
- Get active somewhere that makes you feel good, such as in the park or in a swimming pool.
- Wear clothes that make you feel good and are comfortable.
- Give yourself a specific goal – such as a charity fun run or a 5-a-side friendly. It'll help to keep you focused.
- Be active to music.
- Vary your activity so you don't get bored. For example, if you normally exercise indoors, try an outdoor activity and vice versa.
- Schedule your exercise as if it were an appointment and treat it like one. Write it in your diary and never cancel.

### KEEP YOUR KIDS MOTIVATED
If you find it difficult to get your kids motivated and off the couch, try these ideas. Remember, having fun is the best motivator. And clear evidence of progress will also help everyone to keep going.

- Give kids a sense of achievement – set goals such as beating their previous score.
- Kids love challenges 'against the clock' – use a watch or timer to time them running round the garden or park.
- Keep a chart of achievements.
- Swimming and running clubs' local matches all help to give your kids a focus and something to aim for.

## PLAY TIME

Try something that helps you to discover the big kid inside you. This could be flying a kite, playing Frisbee or using a microscooter. Not all your activities have to be serious or grown-up. Variety is the spice of life!

# Choosing your activities

It's important to choose **activities that you enjoy** and that fit in with your lifestyle. It's no good trying to jog if it leaves you bored senseless. And don't bother to join a club if it takes too much effort to get there regularly. **Be realistic**, start gently and build up gradually over a few months. **That's SAS**!

One of the biggest reasons why people give up exercising is lack of interest. If what you're doing isn't fun, it's hard to keep it up. The good news is there are loads of different activities and sports you can try out to see which one inspires you.

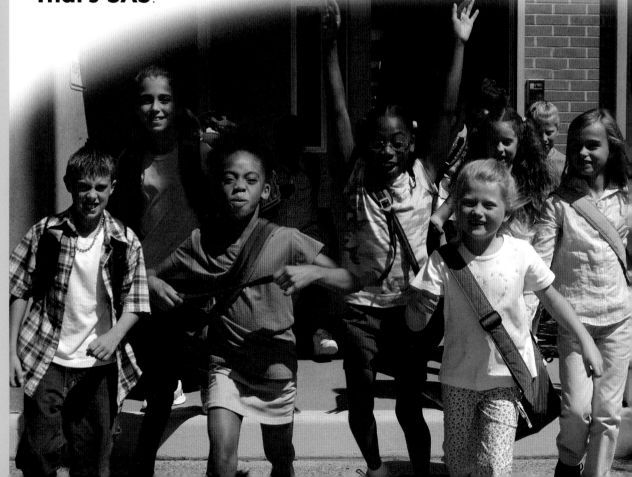

# "If you're not having fun exercising then you're not doing it right!"

**Pregnant**
*It is normally safe to exercise when you are pregnant. Walking, swimming and gentle toning and stretching exercises are best, but check with your GP or midwife first.*

| GOOD FOR | START WITH | ONCE YOU'RE FITTER |
|---|---|---|
| Good for your heart | Walking, cycling, swimming, aqua aerobics | Aerobic/group exercise classes, running, tennis, hockey, circuit training, kick boxing |
| Good for strength | Digging, swimming, hill-walking, beginner pilates classes | Weight training, tubing or resistance bands, circuit training, body-pump classes, pilates, Ashtanga yoga |
| Good for keeping you supple | Stretch classes, beginner yoga classes | Yoga, tai chi, pilates |

IAN WRIGHT'S FITTER FAMILIES

# Exercise in your own time

"But I haven't got time to exercise!" I hear you say. Well, **the good news** is you don't need a lot of time to get fit. Yes, really! There are lots of **simple ways** to incorporate more exercise into your daily routine. You can get **fitter** at home, at work, indoors, outdoors …

### WALKING OFF CALORIES

If you walk for 30 minutes on the flat, at a moderate 5km/h, you'll burn around 160 calories. If you walk a bit quicker, at a brisk 6.5km/h, you'll burn 200 calories. Add some hills and you could burn an extra 100 calories.

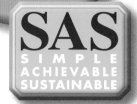

**SAS**
SIMPLE
ACHIEVABLE
SUSTAINABLE

The simplest way to get fit is to walk more. Whether it's taking the kids to school, or walking to work, the simple act of putting one foot in front of the other is a great way to build activity into your day.

### WALK MORE

You can walk anytime, anywhere. It's simple, it's free and it's one of the best ways to get fit. To turn everyday walking into fitness walking, lengthen your stride, quicken your pace, keep going and do it regularly.

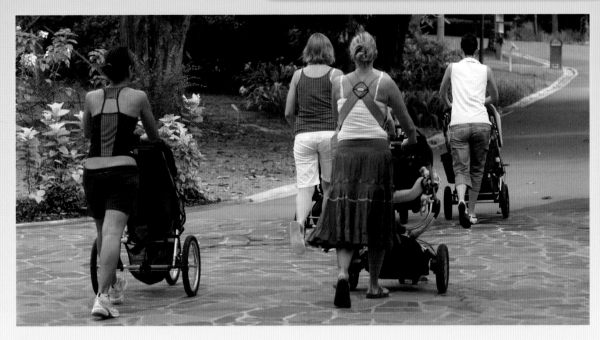

## AT HOME

If you don't fancy going out running or joining an aerobics class, you can still get fitter in your own home. There are dozens of ways to get active without leaving the house. And the good news is that none of them will cost you a penny!

⭐ Put on some music and dance around the house – it's a fantastic and fun way to get fit.

⭐ Get fit while you brush your teeth – stand on your right leg while you brush your teeth with your left hand for a minute. Then swap over. Easy!

⭐ Make housework into a workout. When you vacuum, dust, clean or scrub, do it a bit faster and work up a sweat.

# "A few easy changes a day will help you get fit."

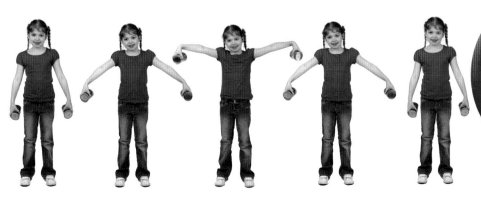

### BE CREATIVE
Got a can of beans? Then you've got a dumbbell. Use the things around your home – it will save you money.

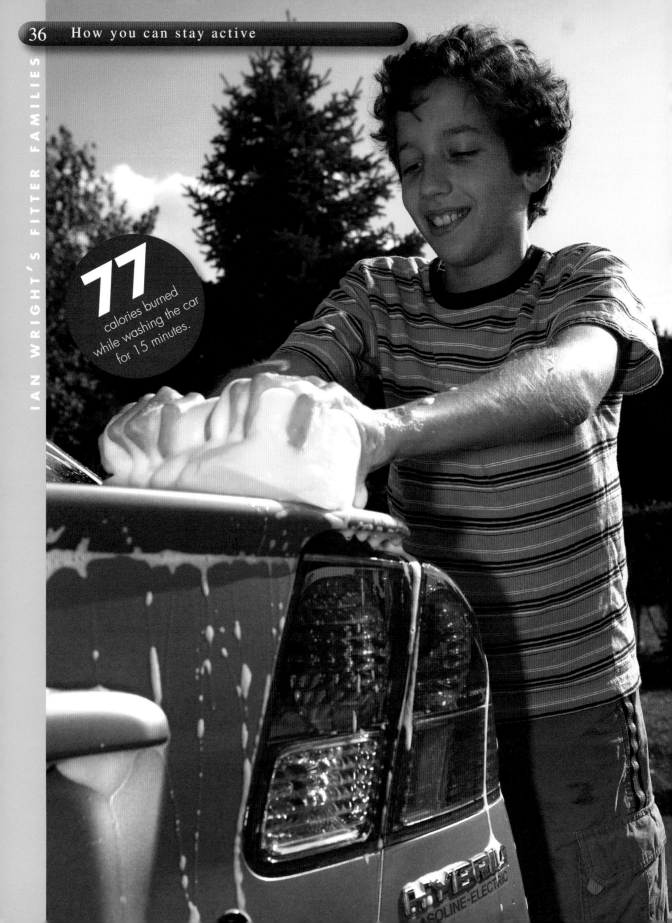

IAN WRIGHT'S FITTER FAMILIES

**77** calories burned while washing the car for 15 minutes.

Everyone needs to spend more time being active and less time in front of the television. But that doesn't mean you need to go to the gym. There are loads of activities to do around the house.

## WHILE WATCHING TV

You don't have to give up your favourite programme to exercise. Here are some ways to get fit during those commercial breaks.

### Step to it

Once the adverts start, walk up and down the stairs once before returning to the TV.

### Push 'n' crunch

Try to do as many push-ups as you can during one advert. For the next advert try to do as many crunches, or sit-ups, as you can. Keep going until the end of the break.

### Happy hearts

Try marching or jogging on the spot. Do some jumping jacks or knee-lifts.

## IN THE GARDEN

Working in the garden, raking leaves, digging – these activities all burn around 350 calories in an hour. They're also great for toning the muscles in your arms, legs, back and stomach. An hour of energetic digging and weeding can burn as many as 500 calories.

**TOP TIP**
There is no 'best way' to get fit. Any movement is good and it doesn't have to be a gym workout. You can fit lots of activity into your life by doing things you enjoy. Dance, ride a bike or take a brisk walk. It all counts. And if you're short of time, break down your daily exercise into ten-minute activities.

**SAS**
SIMPLE
ACHIEVABLE
SUSTAINABLE

**90** calories burned while mowing the lawn for 20 minutes.

**88** calories burned walking briskly for 15 minutes.

# Exercise while you work

Being at work **doesn't mean** you have to sit still all day. From walking to work to **sneaky exercises** by the drinks machine, there are loads of ways to **build exercise into your working day** and get fitter.

**P**ace up and down the platform while waiting for a train. Stand rather than sit on the train – it'll improve your balance and stability. Pull in your stomach muscles gently while you are driving the car. On the bus, always climb to the top deck if there is one – it will give your legs a good workout.

## "Just like any meeting, schedule exercise in your diary."

**TOP TIP**
You won't have time to run a marathon in your lunch break, but a lap of the local park would be a good start.

IAN WRIGHT'S FITTER FAMILIES

# GETTING TO WORK

Don't use the excuse that you can't be active while you travel to work. Just walk further and take the car or public transport less.

### Walk to work

Walk to work or park further from the office. Walk tall, push off from your heels and through your toes and swing your arms. Try to pick up the pace, walking just a bit faster each week.

### Walk up the escalator

Walking up escalators instead of standing still burns around 10 calories per minute and is a great way to tone your bottom and legs. Even walking down escalators burns 4 calories per minute.

### Get off the bus

Get off the bus earlier and walk. Time your walk and, each week, try to beat the previous week's time.

# MAKE YOUR LUNCHTIMES COUNT

Walk somewhere to get lunch or, if you bring in your own sandwiches, walk somewhere to eat them. Even if you only go to the park five minutes away, that's an extra 50 minutes of activity at the end of a working week! Maybe there's a swimming pool close by where you could fit in a 20-minute swim.

# USE THE STAIRS

Use stairs rather than the lift. A few flights a day will tone up your leg muscles and get your heart pumping.

# IN YOUR OFFICE

Use every opportunity to move.

- Rise up on your toes while you're waiting for the photocopier or standing by the drinks machine.
- Do a few shoulder circles while you're sitting at your desk.
- Do a few squats by your desk when the office is quiet.
- Keep moving about when you are on the phone.

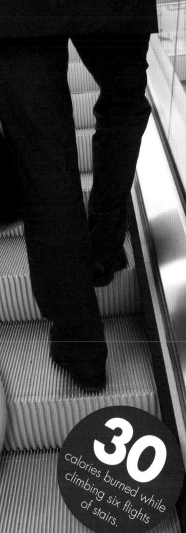

**TOP TIP**
If you have to sit behind a desk at work, make sure you don't slouch in your chair. Sitting with a good posture tones your stomach muscles and helps you to avoid having back problems. Organise your desk so that your keyboard is close to you and the computer screen is level with your eyes.

**30** calories burned while climbing six flights of stairs.

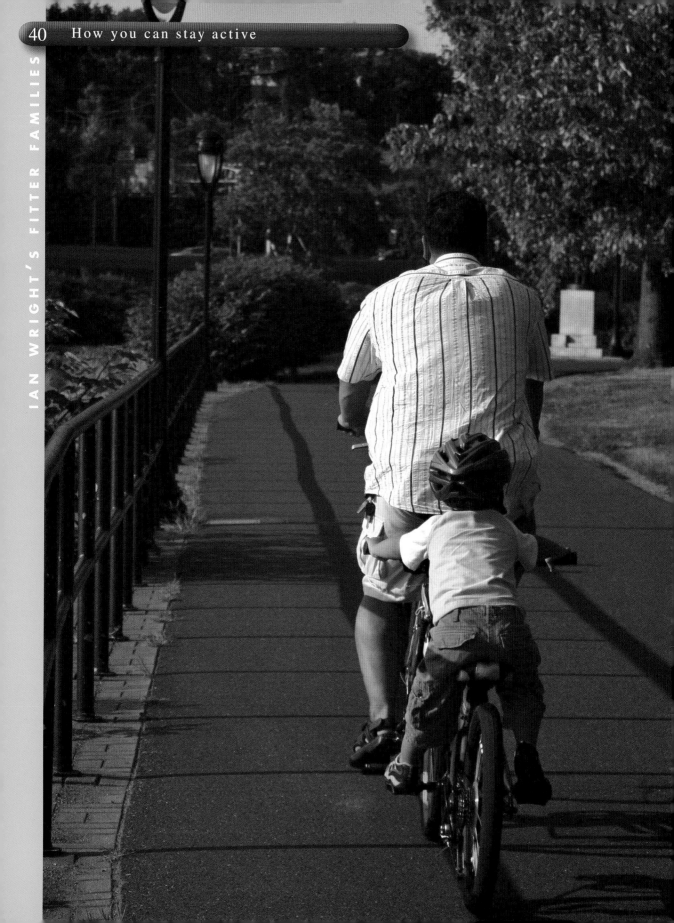

IAN WRIGHT'S FITTER FAMILIES

# Getting around

These days we all seem to lead **hectic lives**. We all think we're **too busy** to fit everything in and that our time gets swallowed up by daily chores, leaving us no **time** to lead a healthier lifestyle. But **it's not true!**

**L**ook for different ways to get around town when you're doing your usual chores. I've already said that walking more and walking faster is a great way to squeeze activity into your day. The same goes for cycling or rollerblading or even riding a microscooter. Are you popping to the shops for a pint of milk, getting the kids to school or heading to the post office? Then leave the car behind. Small journeys in the car are bad for the environment so you can be green and get fit at the same time!

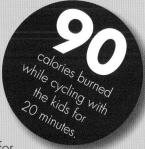

**90** calories burned while cycling with the kids for 20 minutes.

## ANYWHERE AT ALL

There are all kinds of places you can be more active. For example, sometimes you do need to take the car, such as to the supermarket for your weekly shop. You can still squeeze in some extra activity though. Park further away from the supermarket door and return the shopping trolley to the supermarket entrance after getting back to your car. This also saves you the hassle of trying to get one of those popular parking spaces by the door!

## PUSHING A BUGGY

Pushing a pram or buggy briskly around town for 30 minutes is a great workout for busy parents. It tones your legs, bottom, stomach and shoulders. You can also meet other parents this way: log on to www.powerpramming.co.uk for details of powerpramming classes in your area.

> "Use your imagination and your errands turn into free exercise classes!"

**TOP TIPS**
* Where there is a pavement or footpath, use it.
* If there is no pavement, walk on the right-hand side of the road to face the traffic.
* Be safe. Be seen. Wear bright clothing in bad weather or at dusk. Fluorescent materials show up in daylight and dusk. Reflective bands are good at night.

**SAS**
SIMPLE
ACHIEVABLE
SUSTAINABLE

"Make walking a family habit."

# Exercising together

As well as **squeezing in** more activity to your day at the office or while doing your chores, remember to **plan activities** to do together as a family.

### WALK YOUR KIDS TO SCHOOL
Walking first thing wakes up their bodies and brains so they'll have more energy during the day and concentrate better at school. Make sure they wear comfortable shoes with low heels.

### TAKE THEM TO THE LOCAL SWIMMING POOL
Splashing around in the pool with the kids is a great energiser. If you feel uncomfortable in swimming gear at first, remember that you're doing this for yourself. It's not important what anyone else thinks.

- Swimming is good all-round exercise. It uses almost every muscle in the body.
- Enjoy the feeling of being in the water. It doesn't matter how fast you swim at first.
- Try to swim five lengths. Once you can manage that, add another couple of lengths, and so on. Set yourself SAS goals.
- Time your lengths and try to improve your times with each visit.
- Play throwing and catching games if you're allowed to, when the pool isn't busy.

### PLAN A TRIP TO YOUR LOCAL SPORTS CENTRE
Book a badminton or tennis court. You'll have fun while getting a good workout. Find out about dancing, martial arts, gymnastics or football classes for kids.

### FAMILY BIKE RIDE
It could be a simple ride to the park or a longer trip. Pack a picnic and make a day of it. However short the ride, make sure everyone wears a correctly fitting helmet. Take a repair kit for any punctures.

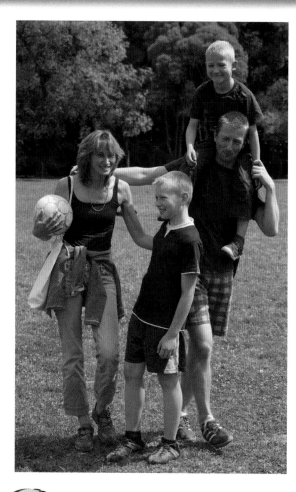

**W**hen I was a kid, my favourite time was always when my friends were around or we were down our local park, running about and playing different games.

### IN THE PARK

You don't need expensive equipment. Run about, kick a ball, skip rope, fly a kite, fling a Frisbee – they're much better value than a pricey visit to the gym.

### FOOTBALL

Football is great for getting kids fit. Running and sprinting for the ball improves stamina. Kicking, tackling and passing are good for balance and coordination. Playing football builds friendships and teaches kids how to work together.

### FRISBEE

This is a fantastic game to play in the garden or park. It'll test your coordination, speed and strength all at once. Make it into a game of piggy-in-the-middle to add a bit of extra competition.

### GAMES

★ Rounders – for six or more of you. All you need is a bat and ball and any handy objects to mark the 'posts'.

★ Hop scotch. Use chalk to mark the grid. Try to be the first to get to the top.

★ Treasure hunt. Ask a friend to hide some 'treasures' in the garden. Run and find them.

Rugby ball

Football

Tennis ball

Frisbee

Soft rubber ball

Different racquets

Skipping rope

**TOP TIPS**

Adventure playgrounds are a fun way to get kids active. Balancing on logs, scrambling over climbing walls, swinging on ropes and skinning up climbing frames will all get kids fit without them noticing it. The activities will also promote sharing and good social skills and are a way to make new friends.

IAN WRIGHT'S FITTER FAMILIES

# Indoor activities

Rainy skies, **snowstorms** and brisk winter temperatures may mean that you have to **stay indoors**. However, being indoors does not mean that you can't be active. **Try these activities** the next time your family is stuck indoors!

**K**eep the activities varied because it keeps the family interested and their bodies challenged. This also gives the family a good understanding of the many different types of sport that are on offer to them and allows them to try new activities that they might never have considered doing before.

### BEANBAG GLUE
Move around the house while balancing a beanbag on various body parts. Young children can try to crawl while balancing the beanbag on their back. Older children can try walking with the beanbag on their head, shoulder or back of the hand while changing directions.

### BOWLERAMA
Place a target, such as plastic cups, at the end of the hallway. Standing at the opposite end of the hall, roll a small ball and try to hit the target.

**Climbing high or diving deep**
*Indoor activities don't have to mean staying at home. Your local sports centre may have a climbing wall or a swimming pool. Try something new — you could discover a hidden talent!*

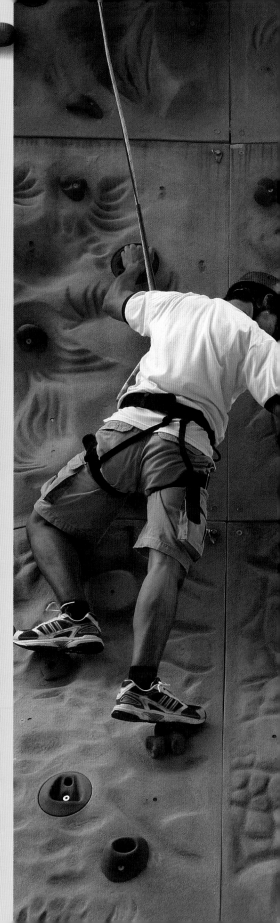

IAN WRIGHT'S FITTER FAMILIES

### ANIMAL CHASE

Try this game at a young child's party. Children form a circle. A teddy or other toy animal is sent around the circle and, while it is going round, another toy is introduced. The object of the game is for the second toy to try to catch up with the first. More toys can be introduced.

"Indoor balloon volleyball can be great fun. Use a table as the net."

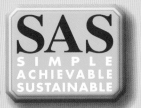

**SAS**

SIMPLE
ACHIEVABLE
SUSTAINABLE

# Ian's family fun

### Frisbee fun

*Once you've mastered the basic skills of throwing a Frisbee, get a couple of families or mates together for a game of Ultimate Frisbee. It's a fantastic team game and really gets your body moving. It's simple – even your kids can play!*

It's important for **everyone in your family** to keep active. You'll all have loads of fun getting fit together. Here are some **fun ideas**. All you need is a ball or a Frisbee, a **bunch of mates** or a couple of families and enough space to run around.

**104** calories burned playing Frisbee for half an hour

### How to play Ultimate Frisbee

The object of the game is to score points by passing the Frisbee into the opponents' end zone, similar to American football. You need two teams with (ideally) seven players in each. To begin the game, Team A throws the Frisbee to Team B, who catch it. Team B's challenge is then to pass the Frisbee between themselves while moving towards their opponents' end zone. They cannot run with the Frisbee. They can only pivot on one foot. Meanwhile, the other team tries to gain possession of the Frisbee by knocking it down etc. They then try to reach the other end zone. A team scores a point when one of the team catches the Frisbee in the opponents' end zone. Whichever team gets the most points by the end of the game wins.

### Keeping fit

*Playing Frisbee keeps me fit. All that zig-zag running and those cutting movements to get to free space develop agility and endurance. And catching the Frisbee develops good hand-eye-disc coordination.*

## Tag rugby

*This is a fun version of non-contact rugby. No tackling, scrums, or line-outs are allowed, so it's perfect for kids! Play it in the park or on the beach, or as a competitive game in organised leagues and festivals. Log on to www.tagrugby.org for more information.*

**297**
calories burned playing tag rugby for half an hour

**Myths**

**FACT:** A 2008 study of 60,000 people in the USA found that those who did moderate rather than excessive exercise had a lower risk of stroke.

**Facts**

IAN WRIGHT'S FITTER FAMILIES

"Make exercise a habit and enjoy doing something active every day."

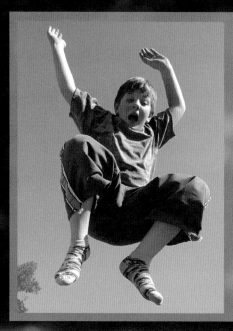

**Try a trampoline**
*Trampolining is good exercise as well as being great fun. Reduce the risk of accidents by ensuring yours has safety pads and a safety net or cage. Always supervise children and don't allow somersaults and stunts. Never allow more than one person on the trampoline at the same time.*

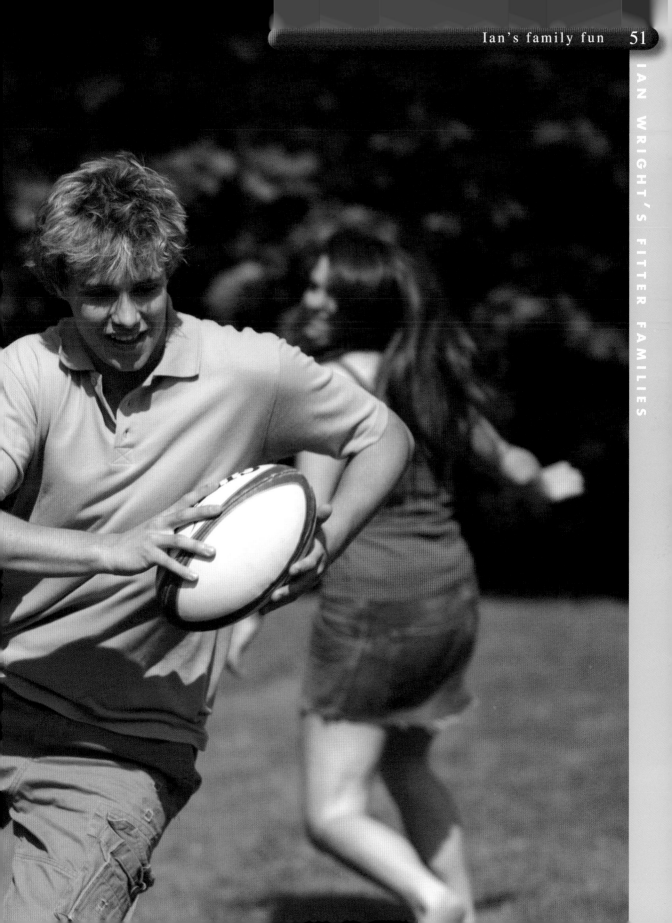

# More family fun

**Use the outdoors** – don't let our British weather stop you getting out with the family. The outdoors will energise you. **Any open space**, whether it's a park, a common or just your garden, offers tons of opportunities for getting active and having fun.

### Swings and ladders
*Outdoor play equipment provides kids with fun, fresh air and exercise. Always supervise young kids and only let them use age-appropriate equipment. Pre-schoolers should climb only 1.5 metres high, school-age kids only 2 metres. Remind kids to bend their knees when they jump to the ground and to land on both feet together.*

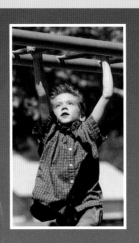

Go on adventure walks with the kids. Even a garden can be an adventure. Use your imagination and it could be a jungle, a circus or even Wembley Stadium.

### TRY YOUR LOCAL FACILITIES
All local authorities provide some form of health and fitness facilities, and while charges vary between councils, many centres have open days when you can use facilities for free to see whether you like them. Have a look at their websites and find out what's on offer in your area. There are also some free basketball, five-a-side and tennis courts around.

### MORE THINGS TO TRY
Still stuck for ideas? How about kite flying – it's a great way to get the family on its feet. A simple one-string kite will keep younger kids happy; a more advanced stunt kite will be challenging for older kids. Or try basketball in your garden – put a hoop on the side of your house and challenge the family to a shootout.

### Tree climbing
*See how high you can climb – but make sure you know the tree is safe for climbing first.*

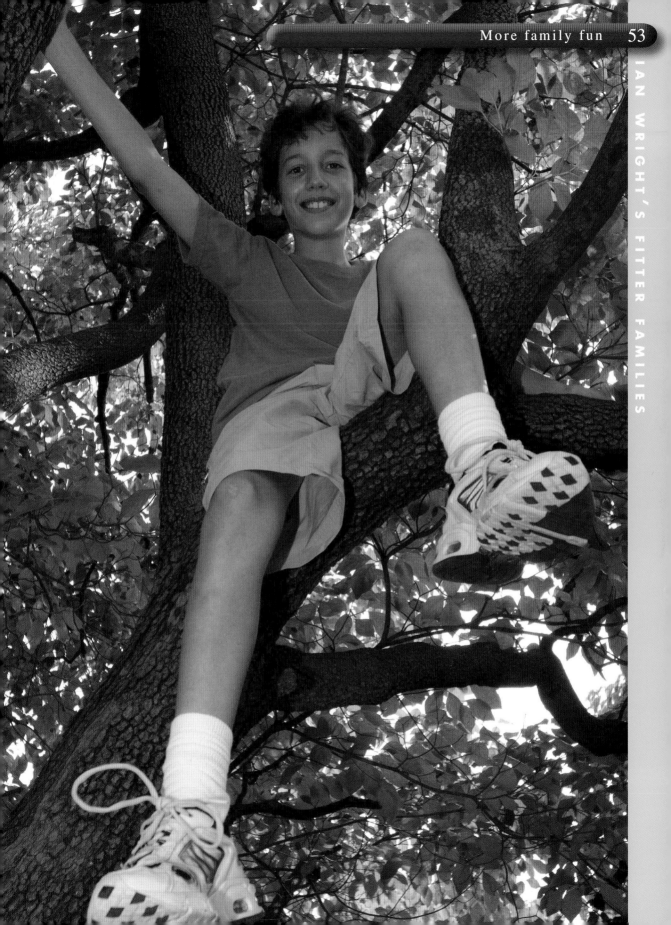

**S**kipping raises your heart rate and your spirits, is a great way to burn calories and can bring back the joys of childhood. All you need is a skipping rope, a pair of trainers and enough space to turn the rope.

## BENEFITS OF SKIPPING

Skipping dramatically improves your balance, coordination and timing. It strengthens legs and the upper body as well as boosting your cardiovascular fitness. It also builds strong bones. You can do it outside in the sunshine or inside if its cold.

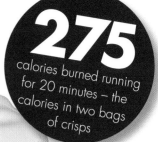

**275** calories burned running for 20 minutes – the calories in two bags of crisps

## Myths & Facts

**FACT:** Skipping at a moderate speed of 70 to 120 turns per minute for 15 minutes burns 150 to 200 calories – as much as running a ten-minute mile.

### Do it right
*Jump just high enough to clear the rope, and land with your knees slightly bent. Transfer your weight from one foot to the other as you skip. Keep the rope close to your head as it swings over you.*

### It's simple
*Jogging is one of the simplest ways to get fit. If you can put one foot in front of the other, you can jog. And you can do it where and when you like.*

# "Playing active games doesn't feel like real exercise – but it is!"

### Play tag
*All you need to play tag is three or more people. Kids or adults can play. One person is 'it', and that person runs around and tries to touch someone else. If they succeed, the person they touch is now 'it' and tries to chase everyone else.*

**206** calories burned playing tennis for 30 minutes

### Have a game of tennis
*Tennis is great for improving your fitness as well as your hand-ball-eye coordination. Many parks have tennis courts that can be hired for a small charge or are even free.*

**SAS**
SIMPLE
ACHIEVABLE
SUSTAINABLE

### TOP TIPS
Holiday sports clubs are great fun. Many offer sports that your kids may not have tried before, such as indoor climbing or dry slope skiing, as well as popular activities such as dance and trampolining.

### Play rounders
*If you're having a family picnic, take a bat and ball for a game of rounders. It's great fun and you'll get fit in no time. You can set up a local league. Log on to www.nra-rounders.co.uk for more information.*

### Winter fun

*Ice skating is an exhilarating winter activity that will help you to develop balance. An hour of leisurely ice skating burns 310 calories, the equivalent of a medium hamburger. Log on to www.iceskatingrinks.net to find your nearest rink.*

# Even more ideas

You can get fitter in **so many ways**. Trying a new sport together can be challenging and rewarding. You may discover **hidden talents** or unleash a healthy competitive streak! Whatever you do, the key is to **make it fun**.

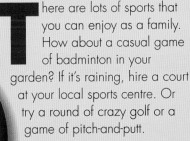

**TOP TIPS**
Indoor climbing can give kids confidence as well as a healthier body and mind. Instead of you against another person, climbing is you against the rock. To be a good climber, you'll need to keep your cool, take your time, and carefully plan your way up.

There are lots of sports that you can enjoy as a family. How about a casual game of badminton in your garden? If it's raining, hire a court at your local sports centre. Or try a round of crazy golf or a game of pitch-and-putt.

## TRY CLIMBING A WALL

There are hundreds of climbing walls in the UK just waiting to be climbed. Climbing works both your upper and lower body muscles and burns 340 calories per half hour. All indoor climbing centres run sessions for beginners and children. Find your nearest climbing wall by visiting www.ukclimbing. com/databases.

## GO SKATING

In-line skating and skateboarding are fun, but make sure you keep away from busy roads and wear pads and helmets. Rollerblade or skateboard only on the pavement, NEVER on the road.

### Skateboarding
*Playgrounds, parks and specially designated areas are the best places to go skateboarding.*

# Safety first

Whether you're **riding your bike** to school, to the local shop or to visit friends, always ride carefully and never take unnecessary risks. You should **always wear a helmet**. Wearing a helmet could prevent concussion, brain damage or even death.

"Always wear safety gear – no matter how cool you think it is to go without."

## HELMETS

Most helmets are made of polystyrene with a plastic and lycra coating and have undergone strict safety tests. Make sure yours fits properly. Test this by putting on the helmet and shaking your head. The helmet should not shift around or fall forwards.

## BEFORE YOU GO

Make sure your bike is the right size. Riding a bike which is too big or too small can affect your balance. Check your brakes and tyre pressure before you set off.

- Dress in comfortable clothes: lightweight clothes are best.
- Wear fluorescent materials in daylight and at dusk and something reflective at night.
- Always wear a cycle helmet – it will help to protect you if you have an accident.
- Check that nothing is preventing you from seeing or hearing other road users clearly.
- Make sure other road users can see you clearly too.

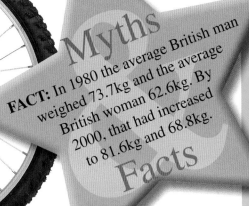

Myths

FACT: In 1980 the average British man weighed 73.7kg and the average British woman 62.6kg. By 2000, that had increased to 81.6kg and 68.8kg.

Facts

# Reward yourself

Rewards can help you to **stay enthusiastic**. They remind you what you've achieved and motivate you to **keep going**. Everyone likes a pat on the back!

**E**veryone should have a reward when they've reached a goal, no matter how small. This could be something as simple as a star or smiley face on your calendar, a relaxing bath or allowing yourself time to read the Sunday papers if you reach your weekly target.

## PLAN AHEAD
Get out the calendar and plan some family outings. Set aside specific times for doing things together, and stick to them! Whether it's a family walk or bike ride, or having a skating session at the leisure centre, it's important to spend active time together.

## NEW ACTIVITIES
See if your family can think of ten fitness activities, then decide which ones you'll have a go at. Do you fancy a game of badminton or some ballroom dancing? Perhaps you fancy a trip to an adventure park. Challenge everyone to try something new.

## FAMILY REWARD
Decide on a reward for the whole family for when it reaches a goal of a certain number of points. Let each family member earn a point for an hour of fitness fun. Rewards could be a trip to a theme park or the cinema.

# and remember ...

- Have fun yourself.
- Smile lots and have a laugh with your family and friends.
- Encourage everyone in the family to feel involved.
- Don't worry if everyone doesn't respond immediately – they may just need more time to warm up.
- Be patient, caring and considerate, and ensure everyone feels they have succeeded.
- Try to finish a game or activity on a high.
- Don't let anyone become bored with the activity before you change it.

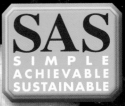

**SAS**
SIMPLE
ACHIEVABLE
SUSTAINABLE

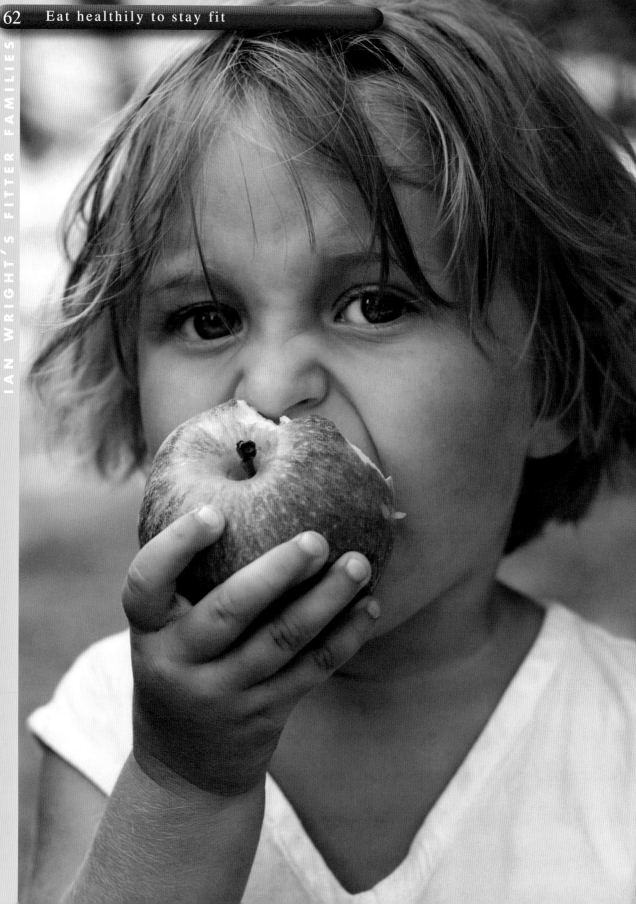

# Eat healthily to stay fit

Now you've set your goals and started to get more active, it's a good idea to **look at what you're eating**. I'm not asking you to go on a diet. In my experience, diets don't work. But I do believe that healthy eating is **important** – you need to fuel your body properly to be fit. You can make small changes to your diet and achieve **big results**.

*Myths & Facts*

**FACT:** Almost one in four British adults are obese, and if current trends continue, 60% of men and 50% of women will be clinically obese by 2050.

# Small steps to good habits

You can still eat your **favourite foods** – just a bit less of some of them and more of other foods! You don't have to eat less, **just better**. Healthy eating is **all about balance** and eating a **variety of foods**. A few small changes to your diet can make all the difference.

E veryone in the family will benefit from a healthier way of eating. It will make you all feel better and look better. Your kids will feel bright and alert and be able to concentrate better at school. They'll suffer fewer illnesses and have plenty of energy. Now that's a good thing!

**Got a sweet tooth?**
*Allow yourself something sweet for each meal, such as a fruit mousse, a handful of sweet grapes or a couple of squares of chocolate. Eat them as part of your meal and you won't get the rollercoaster of energy highs and lows.*

## A LITTLE OF WHAT YOU FANCY

A little of what you fancy is good. If you try to ban a particular food, you'll only end up craving it. As soon as you put something on the forbidden list it becomes the food you absolutely crave.

- You can still eat chocolate – just be sensible about it.
- Schedule a treat into your day – if you know you're allowed a biscuit later, you'll look forward to eating it and you'll stop at one!
- Try the 80/20 rule – if you eat a balanced diet 80% of the time, then you can enjoy other foods you want the other 20% of the time.

## SMALL STEPS

It's not easy trying to give up old unhealthy habits. But if you make one change at a time then it won't feel so hard. Go slowly and make one simple change a week. Your new healthy habits will soon add up and you'll quickly feel the benefits. That's the SAS approach!

- Swap one doughnut for a piece of fruit.
- Have one less takeaway each week.
- Cut down on the sugar in your tea and coffee.
- Instead of chips, have a jacket potato.
- Stop adding salt to your food.

# "Eating healthy food makes me feel better."

## TOP TIPS FOR HEALTHY EATING

Aim for five portions of fruit and veg a day.

Swap sugary and fizzy drinks for water or low-sugar versions.

Always eat food sitting at a table. Eat slowly and enjoy each mouthful.

Drink at least six glasses of water a day.

## SAS
SIMPLE
ACHIEVABLE
SUSTAINABLE

# What about my weight?

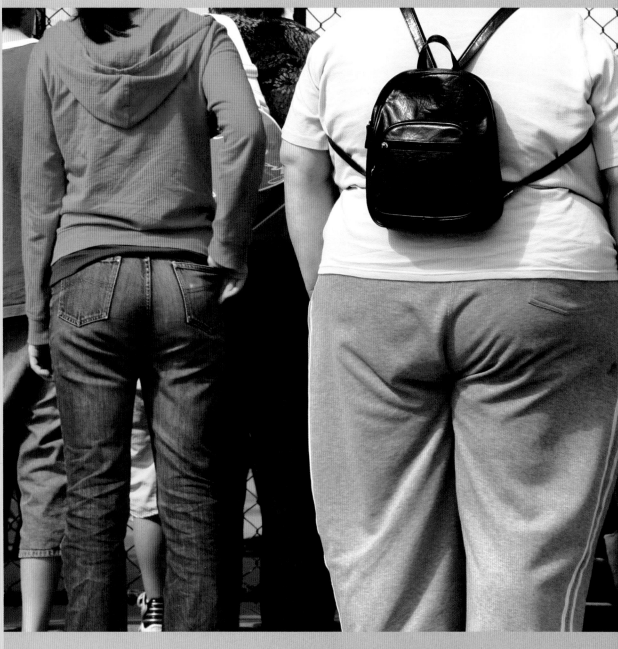

IAN WRIGHT'S FITTER FAMILIES

I don't believe in dieting. Diets might make you lose a bit of weight, but once you come off them, the weight just piles back on again. **Dieting isn't sustainable**. But if you just make small changes to the way you eat and combine that with regular activity, you'll lose weight and **keep it off**. It's a guaranteed way to get you feeling and looking more healthy.

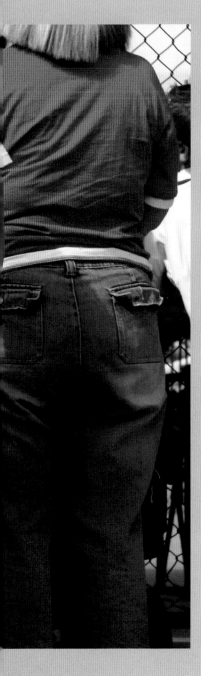

eight loss and gain isn't rocket science. When we take in more calories than we need, we gain weight. But when we use up more calories than we eat, we lose weight. It's as simple as that.

### THE SAS WAY TO LOSE WEIGHT
Losing between 500g and 1kg a week is a healthy and sustainable rate of weight loss. Achieve this by foregoing a couple of biscuits, drinking one less pint of beer and walking an extra half an hour a day. That's a daily saving of 500 calories. Simple!

### LIGHTEN THE LOAD
Drastic calorie chopping can make you lethargic and weak and lead to your body hoarding rather than burning fat. With a sensible eating plan, though, you can lose weight and get fitter.

- Don't nosh while you watch TV – you're more likely to overeat when distracted.
- Say no to seconds – stick to single servings.
- Avoid temptation – buy fruit and veg instead of sugary snacks.
- Use a smaller plate – you'll eat less without noticing.

### CALORIE COUNTING

If you ate one portion of cod and chips – a hefty 753 calories – you would have to do the following to burn off the flab:

1 hour 9 minutes playing football
1 hour 16 minutes cycling
3 hours 38 minutes playing Frisbee
1 hour 49 minutes swimming

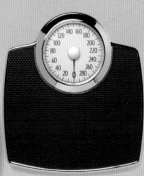

# Six weeks to a healthier you

When it comes to **healthy eating**, you can't expect to overhaul your diet in one week. **If you try to change** everything in one go, your body will rebel and you'll end up scoffing burgers and cakes. Instead, take it **one step** at a time and the changes will feel **achievable** and sustainable.

I t's much easier to replace bad habits with good ones if you take small steps. Make small, simple changes over six weeks and you'll lose those extra kilos for good. Each week, incorporate a new good habit and in six weeks you'll have achieved a big result.

### KEEP A FOOD DIARY

Most of us underestimate how much we eat. But keeping a food diary will make you more aware of what you're eating every day and will show you where the unwanted calories are coming from. Be honest – every handful of crisps and sip of beer counts.

⭐ Write down everything you eat and drink for three days.
⭐ Include every meal, snack and drink that passes your lips.
⭐ Make a note of the amounts – spoonfuls, cups or weight.
⭐ Notice if you are eating too much of something or not enough.
⭐ Work out the changes you could make.

**TOP TIPS FOR HEALTHY EATING**
One simple change can give big results. Cut out one pint of beer a day (300 calories) and you'll lose 12kg in a year.

## "Writing down what you eat makes you think twice before putting it in your mouth!"

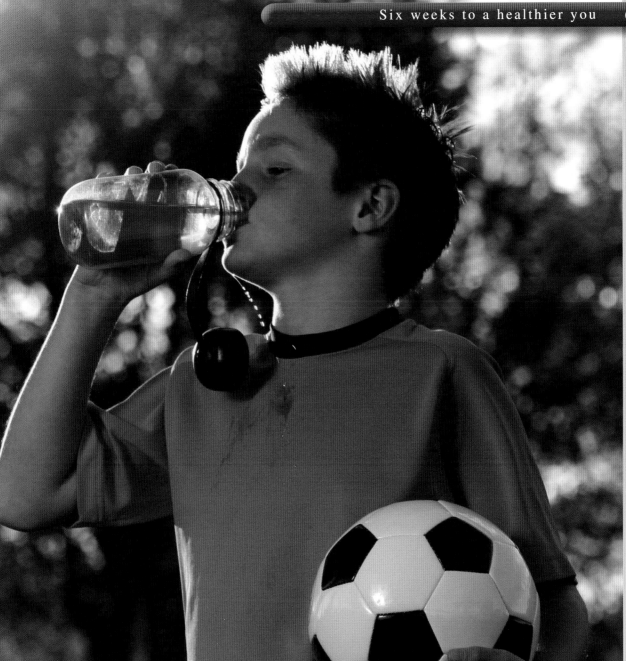

| **WEEK 1** | Swap one can of fizzy drink for a glass of water. |
|---|---|
| **WEEK 2** | Eat an extra piece of fruit each day – try grapes, melon, plums or pears. |
| **WEEK 3** | Eat at least one vegetable at each main meal. |
| **WEEK 4** | Eat one portion of oily fish (sardines, pilchards, salmon) a week. |
| **WEEK 5** | Alternate your usual alcoholic drink with a glass of water. |
| **WEEK 6** | Change your cooking methods – grill, steam or stir-fry food rather than fry it. |

**TOP TIPS**
Stop dieting and let your children see that you enjoy healthy food and regular exercise. Share mealtimes as often as possible and eat the same foods. Don't weigh yourself every day and don't let your children see you on the scales.

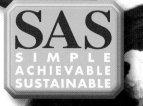

**SAS**
SIMPLE
ACHIEVABLE
SUSTAINABLE

# Eating the right way

Diets are a **short-term fix**. They don't work in the long term. Most are gimmicks and require you to make **too many big changes** to your usual eating habits. The problem is that most people don't like giving up their **favourite foods**. So they **slip up** and go back to their old ways.

## WHAT DOES WORK INSTEAD?

The key to losing weight is to fill up on low-fat, high-fibre foods. That way you won't feel like you're eating less and you won't go hungry. The best appetite-curbing foods are fruit, veg, beans, fish and whole grains.

| EAT THESE | REDUCE THESE |
| --- | --- |
| Wholemeal toast | Chocolate biscuits |
| Slices of apple | Sweets |
| Low-fat yoghurt | Cakes |
| Rice cakes | Crisps |
| Bananas | Chocolate bars |

- Do a mid-way meal check – if you're full, don't feel you have to finish every last morsel.
- Eat your food slowly – it will curb your desire to eat more than you need.
- Plan your day's meals – don't rely on unhealthy snacks and takeaways.
- Don't even think about skipping breakfast.
- Curb evening nibbling – do something active instead!

## CHOOSE FILLING, HEALTHY FOOD

If you eat mostly foods that are nutritious and satisfy your hunger, you will feel full on fewer calories. Feeling full and satisfied while eating foods you like makes it much easier to lose those unwanted kilos.

- Fill up with soup like vegetable soup – it's been proven to make you eat fewer calories.
- Start meals with a salad – but don't use too much dressing.
- Aim to fill half your plate with veg.
- Downsize, not supersize – try to eat only as much as your body really needs.
- Snack on fresh fruit.

IAN WRIG TER FAMILIES

You don't have to eat like a saint all the time. The **key** to achieving and keeping a healthy weight is eating **smaller portions** of foods that are high in sugar, fat and salt.

Myths

**FACT:** One in four 4- to 5-year-olds and almost a third of 10-year-olds are overweight or obese. They face a five times higher risk of being fat as teenagers.

Facts

"Some of these are OK in small amounts, so treat yourself occasionally."

# Try to cut down on these ...

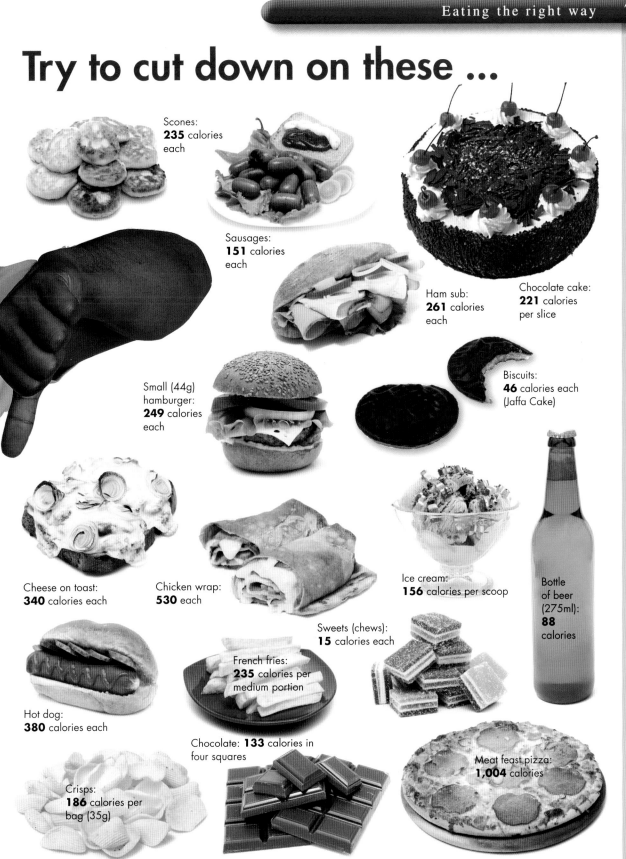

Scones: **235** calories each

Sausages: **151** calories each

Ham sub: **261** calories each

Chocolate cake: **221** calories per slice

Small (44g) hamburger: **249** calories each

Biscuits: **46** calories each (Jaffa Cake)

Cheese on toast: **340** calories each

Chicken wrap: **530** each

Ice cream: **156** calories per scoop

Bottle of beer (275ml): **88** calories

Hot dog: **380** calories each

French fries: **235** calories per medium portion

Sweets (chews): **15** calories each

Chocolate: **133** calories in four squares

Meat feast pizza: **1,004** calories

Crisps: **186** calories per bag (35g)

IAN WRIGHT'S FITTER FAMILIES

# But eat plenty of these ...

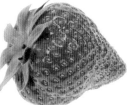

Strawberry:
**73** calories each

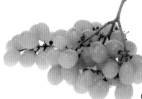

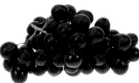

Grapes:
**60** calories per portion

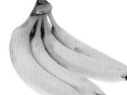

Banana:
**95** calories each

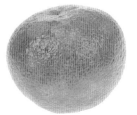

Satsuma:
**25** calories each

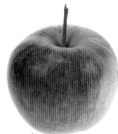

Apple:
**45** calories each

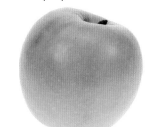

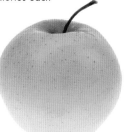

## VEGETABLES
(calories per portion):
Pepper **24** (each)
Tomato **14** (each)
Garlic **3**
Onion **55**
Carrots **15**
Leaf salad **9**
Runner beans **16**
Cabbage **15**
Sweetcorn **100**
Cauliflower **25**
Broccoli **20**
Parsnips **43**
Cucumber **2**
Peas **48**

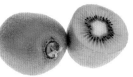

Kiwi fruit:
**30** calories each

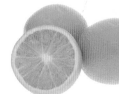

Orange:
**60** calories each

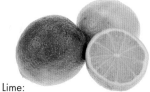

Lime:
**18** calories each

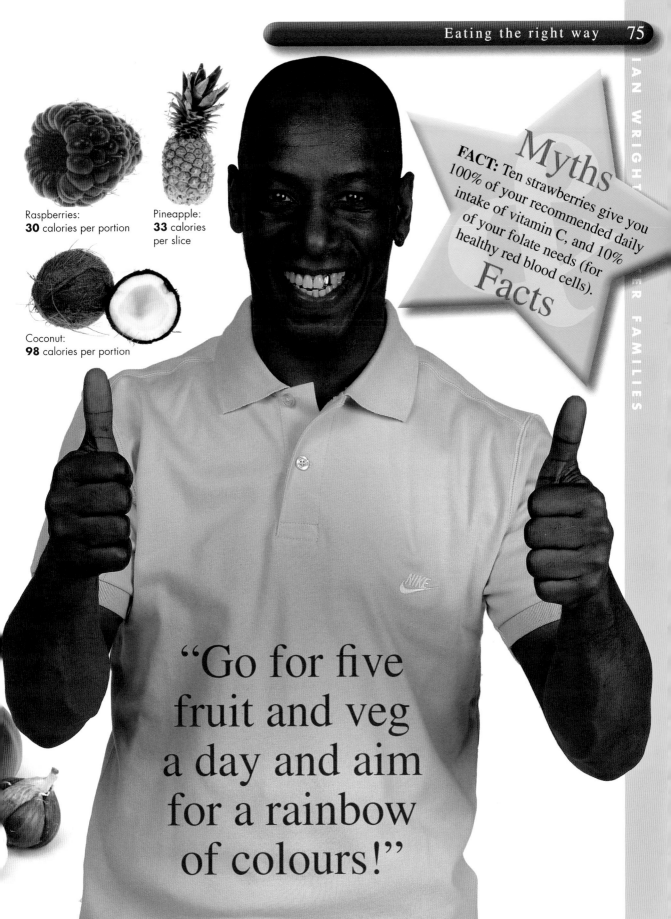

Raspberries:
**30** calories per portion

Pineapple:
**33** calories per slice

Coconut:
**98** calories per portion

## Myths & Facts

**FACT:** Ten strawberries give you 100% of your recommended daily intake of vitamin C, and 10% of your folate needs (for healthy red blood cells).

IAN WRIGHT FAMILIES

"Go for five fruit and veg a day and aim for a rainbow of colours!"

IAN WRIGHT'S FITTER FAMILIES

# Trim the fat

Cutting down the fat in your diet will **help you** to **shed pounds**. Fat provides a lot of calories for very little filling power: 9 calories per gram. This is **more than twice as much** as carbohydrate or protein (4 calories per gram).

**TOP TIPS FOR HEALTHY EATING**
Eat one less ice cream a week and you'll lose more than 1 kilo in a year. An ice cream contains 10g fat – that's two teaspoons.

| INSTEAD OF | EAT SOME |
| --- | --- |
| Burgers, sausages | Lean meat, chicken, fish |
| Biscuits | Cereal bar |
| Crisps | Rice cakes |
| Cake | Plain popcorn |
| Sweets | Fresh or dried fruit |
| Ice cream | Fruit yoghurt |

"I don't fry my food, I grill or bake it whenever I can."

The average man shouldn't eat more than 95g of fat a day; the average women no more than 70g. Try to cut down on 'bad' fats – saturated fats and hydrogenated fats. Both raise the level of cholesterol in your blood and increase your chances of a heart attack.

## AVOID THE BADDIES

Saturated fat is hidden in sausages, burgers, meat, pies and cakes. Hydrogenated fats may be found in biscuits, desserts, ice cream and chocolate bars. Keep these foods for occasional treats only.

- Use semi-skimmed or skimmed milk, not full-fat.
- Use olive oil for cooking and salad dressings.
- Eat fresh fruit instead of desserts and cakes.
- Limit frying except stir-frying using minimal oil.
- Add flavour with fat-free condiments, such as mustard, herbs, soy sauce and salsa.

| GOOD FATS | BAD FATS |
| --- | --- |
| Monosaturated fats: nuts, olive oil, rapeseed oil, avocados, peanut butter | Saturated fats: fatty meats, burgers, sausages, butter, biscuits, cakes, cheese |
| Polyunsaturated fats: nuts, sunflower oil, corn oil, sunflower margarine, seeds | Trans fats: some margarines and spreads, biscuits, pies, cakes, takeaway fried food |
| Omega-3 fats: sardines, salmon, mackerel, pilchards walnuts, omega-3 eggs | |

**Make pizzas healthier**
*Opt for a thin base and extra veggie toppings – tomatoes, peppers, mushrooms and spinach. Delicious!*

*IAN WRIGHT'S FITTER FAMILIES*

# Cut down on the sugar

Sugar is **pure calories**. It makes things **taste sweet** but it provides you with no other goodness. If you're serious about getting into shape, **try to cut down** on the sugar in your diet. It's **not as hard as you might think**.

| AGE | GDA (guideline daily amount) |
|---|---|
| 4–6 years | 40g (2.5 tablespoons) |
| 7–10 years | 50g (3 tablespoons) |
| 11–14 years | 50g (3 tablespoons) |
| 15–18 years | 60g (4 tablespoons) |
| Adult | 60g (4 tablespoons) |

**Heaps of sugar**
*If you have two teaspoons of sugar in your cuppa and you have four cups of tea a day, that's eight teaspoons a day. Put another way, that's 56 teaspoons a week!*

Sugar is bad news for kids. It rots their teeth. Whether it's in sweets, biscuits or sweet drinks, sugar is the major cause of tooth decay. If kids must have sweet things, confine these to mealtimes when they'll do less damage.

## SWEET SECRETS

Sugar doesn't just come from obvious foods such as chocolate and cakes. Breakfast cereals, sauces, cereal bars and fruit bars contain lots of hidden sugar too. Check the label for words such as sucrose, glucose syrup, invert sugar and glucose – they're all forms of added sugar.

## CUTTING DOWN

Adults should have no more than 60g added sugar a day, children no more than 50g. We should eat foods that provide us with energy and other nutrients. Go for fresh fruit, dried fruit, smoothies and fruit juice.

⭐ Scrutinise labels. Opt for foods containing less than 5g sugar per 100g (these may have green traffic light labels). Avoid anything with more than 15g per 100g (red traffic light labels).

⭐ Cut down on the amount of sugar you take in coffee and tea.

⭐ Swap snack bars that are high in sugar for fruit.

⭐ Opt for breakfast cereals with no or little sugar, such as Shreddies, Weetabix or porridge.

"Check your labels – sometimes 'health food' isn't as healthy as it sounds."

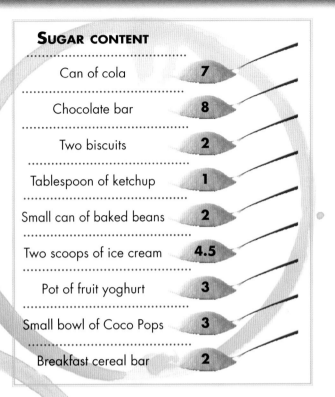

**SUGAR CONTENT**

| | |
|---|---|
| Can of cola | 7 |
| Chocolate bar | 8 |
| Two biscuits | 2 |
| Tablespoon of ketchup | 1 |
| Small can of baked beans | 2 |
| Two scoops of ice cream | 4.5 |
| Pot of fruit yoghurt | 3 |
| Small bowl of Coco Pops | 3 |
| Breakfast cereal bar | 2 |

**TOP TIP**
Be careful! Many fruit products aimed at children, such as fruit bars, claim 'no added sugar' but contain concentrated fruit puree and juice. These are as bad for kids as ordinary sugar.

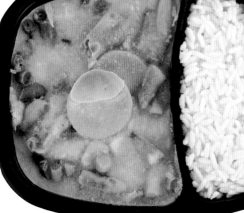

**WARNING!**
A cheeseburger with a small portion of fries contains 3.3g salt. This is more than a young child's daily maximum intake, and more than half an adult's.

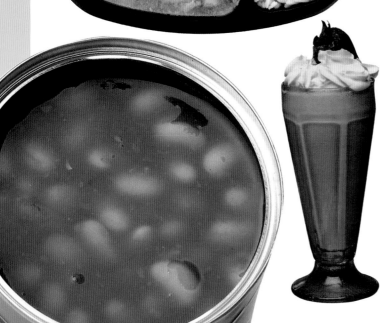

| TYPICAL SALT CONTENT | |
| --- | --- |
| Bowl of Frosties | **1.5g** |
| Pizza | **1.3g** |
| Beefburger | **2.0g** |
| Sausage | **1.2g** |
| Crisps | **0.6g** |
| Ready meal | **1.9g** |
| Mllk shake | **0.5g** |
| Small can of beans | **2.5g** |
| Two fish fingers | **1.3g** |
| Pasta sauce | **1.0g** |
| Chicken nuggets | **1.8g** |

# Eat less salt

A small amount of salt is essential for keeping you healthy. But **too much** salt leads to raised **blood pressure** and increases the risk of a **heart attack** or **stroke**. The chances are you are eating more than you need.

It's important to keep an eye on how much salt the whole family is consuming. Children are particularly vulnerable to the effects of salt but, despite requiring less salt than adults, the average child in the UK consumes as much as 10 to 12g a day.

## HOW MUCH?

Try to limit your daily salt intake to 6g. Children under 7 should have no more than 3g of salt a day. Those between 7 and 10 should have no more than 5g a day and those aged 11+ should have no more than 6g.

## WATCH OUT FOR HIDDEN SALT

Three-quarters of the salt we eat comes from processed food, so you may not realise how much salt you and your kids are eating. Meat products (ham, bacon, sausages and burgers), bread, soups, sauces, cheese, ready meals, pizzas, baked beans, breakfast cereals and biscuits can all be high in salt.

⭐ Cut down on tinned foods, such as pasta shapes in tomato sauce and baked beans.
⭐ Eat fewer burgers, sausages and chicken nuggets.
⭐ Swap salty snacks like crisps for unsalted nuts, plain popcorn, dried fruit, grapes and satsumas.
⭐ Cut down on ready meals, takeaways and ready-made sauces.

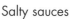

**Salty sauces**
*Go easy with ketchup and mayonnaise – these are very high in salt. Check food labels to find products with less salt and try to stick to the guideline daily amount.*

| AGE | GDA (guideline daily amount) |
|-----|------------------------------|
| 4–6 years | 3g (0.5 teaspoon) |
| 7–10 years | 5g (1 teaspoon) |
| 11–14 years | 6g (just over 1 teaspoon) |
| 15–18 years | 6g (just over 1 teaspoon) |
| Adult | 6g (just over 1 teaspoon) |

**WARNING!**
Eating lots of salt causes high blood pressure, which triples the risk of you having heart disease or a stroke. Cut down on salt and reduce your blood pressure.

# What your body needs

Eating a **healthy diet** isn't as complicated as you may think. You need to **balance** the energy (calories) you consume with the energy you burn. Aim to eat a **wide variety** of foods from each of the major food groups and you should get all the essential **nutrients** your body needs.

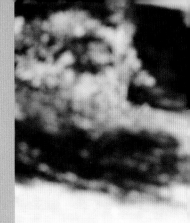

**A good start**
*Share mealtimes when you can. If children learn to enjoy a balanced diet now, they'll continue to eat well and stay healthy as they get older.*

**E**ach day your body needs carbohydrates, fats, proteins, vitamins minerals and water.

### CARBOHYDRATES

Carbohydrates include sugars and starch and are your main source of energy. They fuel your muscles as well as your brain and other organs. Aim to have six portions of starchy carbohydrates a day. At least three of these should be wholegrain – more if you are very active. Good sources of carbohydrate include:

- Wholemeal bread
- Wholegrain breakfast cereals, e.g. porridge, Bran Flakes, Weetabix, Shredded Wheat
- Pasta and rice
- Potatoes and parsnips
- Beans and lentils
- Sweetcorn and peas

### FATS

You need a little fat for energy and for making healthy body cells. Make sure you choose 'good' fats (see page 76). Fats also supply vitamins A, D and E. Try these:

- Olive and other vegetable oils
- Vegetable oil margarine
- Oily fish such as mackerel
- Avocados
- Nuts and seeds

### PROTEINS

You need protein for growth and repairing body cells, as well as for making enzymes and hormones. Aim to eat two or three portions of any of the following each day:

- Meat, chicken, turkey, fish
- Milk, cheese, yoghurt
- Eggs
- Beans and lentils
- Nuts and seeds
- Soya and quorn

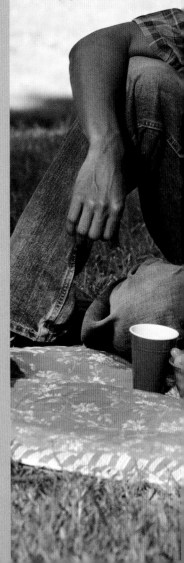

## Myths & Facts

**MYTH**: It's a myth that children grow out of unhealthy eating habits. They go on eating the foods they're used to, so need healthy habits when they're young.

## TOP TIPS

Encourage kids to drink water by adding slices of lemon or lime or frozen cubes of fruit juice. Give them a novelty water bottle. And set a healthy example – drink water yourself.

## FRUIT AND VEG

*Prepare fruit and veg properly so that they retain their nutrients.*

⭐ *Buy fresh-looking, unblemished fruit and veg or use frozen, which is speedily processed and retains its vitamins.*

⭐ *Prepare fruit and veg just before use. They lose their nutrients once cut.*

⭐ *Steam or boil veg in the minimum of water to preserve their vitamins.*

⭐ *Add veg to fast-boiling water. Cook briefly until tender-crisp.*

Physical activity requires the **right fuel**. That's why it's important to eat a wide variety of fresh, nutritious foods. Ensure your meals combine **carbohydrates**, moderate amounts of **protein** – and **fruit and vegetables** of course. The whole family will have bags of energy!

Look at nutrient information on food packages to help you make healthier choices. Some foods have traffic light labels on the front of the pack. These tell you whether the food has high, medium or low amounts of things you should avoid – fats, salt and sugar. Aim to buy mostly greens and fewer reds.

## VITAMINS AND MINERALS

Your body needs vitamins and minerals to keep healthy and fight illnesses. All have a special role to play. They are vital for kids' growth and development. On the whole, the body can't make vitamins and minerals. That's where food comes in.

## WATER

Water really is important. It makes up around 60% of our bodies. If you don't drink enough you may get a headache, be unable to concentrate properly and feel tired more quickly. You should try to drink at least six cups or glasses of water a day, and more in hot weather and during exercise. Carry a bottle of water with you through the day and keep one on your desk at work. Drink plenty of water before, during and after exercise.

**Full of goodness**
*Fruit and veg are rich in vitamin C and are a great source of fibre. They also provide antioxidants for a healthy immune system.*

IAN WRIGHT'S FITTER FAMILIES

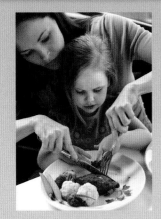

**A bit of encouragement**
*Get your kids to try a new vegetable by mixing it with a food they already like.*

**TOP TIP**
Jazz up vegetables with grated cheese, tomato ketchup or tasty sauce. Broccoli, cauliflower and brussels sprouts go well with cheese sauce; beans, peas and sweetcorn can be put into pasta sauce.

# Five a day

One of the **easiest and tastiest** ways to stay healthy is to eat plenty of **fruit and vegetables**. Try to eat 5 a day and aim to eat a variety of **different colours**: orange, red, green, purple, white, yellow. Each gives you different **health benefits**.

High levels of fruit and veg boost immunity, making you less likely to get colds and flu, especially if you eat fruit and veg rich in vitamin C, such as satsumas, oranges, kiwi fruit, strawberries, red peppers and cabbage. They're all delicious! 5 a day protects against many cancers in later life. It also helps cut the risk of heart disease and stroke. You may have to be determined and sometimes sneaky to get kids to eat their fruit and veg. Give them fresh or dried fruit as snacks. Put the fruit bowl within easy reach of little hands!

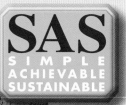

**SAS**
SIMPLE
ACHIEVABLE
SUSTAINABLE

**FACT:** Potatoes don't count towards the '5 a day' target for fruit and vegetables – they count as starchy, carbohydrate foods.

*Myths & Facts*

## WHAT'S A PORTION?

Here's a guide for adults – for children, portions will be smaller.

### Fruit

⭐ Small fruits – 2 plums, 2 apricots, 2 kiwi fruit, 2 satsumas, 8 strawberries, 12 grapes

⭐ Medium fruits – 1 apple, 1 pear, 1 banana, 1 orange

⭐ Large fruits – half a grapefruit, 5cm slice of melon

⭐ Fruit juice or smoothies – these are one portion, no matter how much you drink.

### Vegetables

⭐ 3 heaped tablespoons of carrots or peas

⭐ 3 broccoli spears

⭐ 5 cherry tomatoes

⭐ 1 small bowl of salad

## IDEAS FOR GETTING ALL FIVE

You can count all the vegetables you put into a casserole or stew. Put plenty of vegetables on home-made pizzas and make soups with vegetables. Try making healthy fruit bars with dried and fresh fruits and oats, and make some healthy biscuits with fruit. In summer you could make ice-lollies and sorbets from fresh fruit.

**A portion of fruit or veg**
*A portion is roughly the amount you can hold in your hand. Children have smaller hands so their portions are smaller and will grow as they grow.*

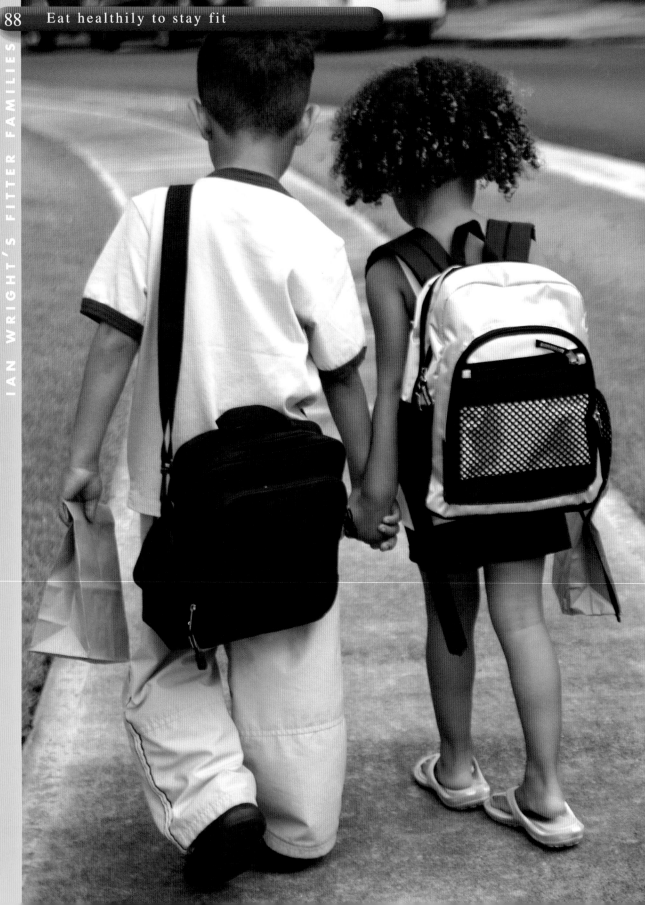

# What's in your lunchbox today?

The **main** things to remember when making a packed lunch are that it is **healthy**, enjoyable, filling and will provide enough **energy** to **sustain** you or your little ones for several hours. It **doesn't have to** break the bank.

T he key to keeping children interested in lunch is variety. Avoid basic sandwiches every day, but keep unhealthy salty or sugary treats, such as crisps, to a minimum.

### THE IDEAL LUNCHBOX

Here is a guide to what your kids should look forward to at lunchtime every day ...

| Day | Lunchbox |
| --- | --- |
| Monday | Wholemeal chicken and tomato sandwich; fruit yoghurt; carrot sticks; satsuma; apple juice |
| Tuesday | Veg soup; wholemeal roll and butter; dried fruit; cheese; yoghurt drink |
| Wednesday | Pizza; strips of pepper or some cherry tomatoes; grapes; yoghurt drink |
| Thursday | Pasta, tuna and mushroom salad; fruit yoghurt; dried apricots; apple juice |
| Friday | Tortilla wrap with turkey and coleslaw; tinned fruit in natural juice with no added sugar; cheese |

⭐ A bottle of water or fruit juice
⭐ A portion of fresh or dried fruit
⭐ Some veg – carrot sticks, or put cucumber or salad in a sandwich with a low-fat dip or dressing
⭐ A sandwich or roll (ideally wholemeal) – filled with chicken, tuna, peanut butter, cheese or egg
⭐ Dairy product – cheese, yoghurt or a milk drink

And try some of these ...

⭐ Pizza slices
⭐ Pasta, potato or rice salad
⭐ Soup in a flask
⭐ Tortilla wraps with interesting fillings
⭐ Oatmeal cookies

# Healthy store cupboard

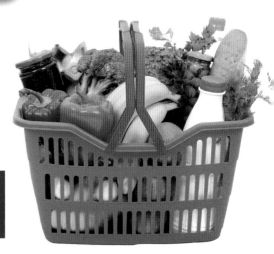

It's **easy** to **whip up** a **healthy meal** if you have the ingredients. You'll be less **tempted** to grab a ready meal or order a takeaway. Next time you shop, take this list of **store cupboard basics**.

There are loads of simple, healthy, cheap and delicious ingredients you can keep around the kitchen. Add them to meals to make sure the whole family is getting their all-important vitamins and minerals.

"Always make sure your fridge is stocked with fresh fruit and veg."

### THE STORE CUPBOARD

Keep these things in your kitchen cupboard to help with healthy meals.

- Tinned tomatoes, baked beans, red kidney beans
- Tinned tuna, sardines, salmon
- Lentils
- Tinned fruit in juice
- Honey
- Pasta and rice
- Olive oil

### FRIDGE OR FREEZER

Stick these foods in your fridge or freezer for delicious and nutritious mealtimes.

- Fresh vegetables
- Fresh fruit
- Fruit juices
- Eggs
- Low-fat milk
- Fresh chicken and lean meat
- Frozen vegetables
- Frozen chicken
- Frozen fish

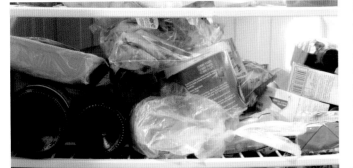

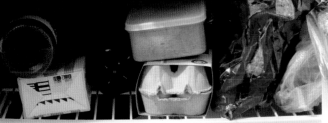

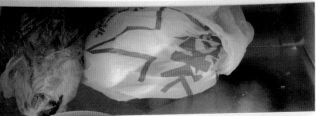

## Food storage
*Store food carefully so that it is safe to eat. Keep food with a use-by date, cooked foods and ready-to-eat foods in the fridge.*

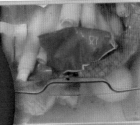

### OMEGA 3s
These essential fats help to protect you against heart disease and stroke, and promote brain development and normal eyesight in children. Oily fish like sardines, salmon and pilchards are packed with them. Try to eat some once a week. Tinned tuna doesn't count because it loses most of its oils in tinning.

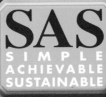

**SAS**
SIMPLE
ACHIEVABLE
SUSTAINABLE

# Start with breakfast

Breakfast is the most **important meal** of the day. When you have a healthy breakfast, you increase your chances of eating healthily throughout the day. You also **fuel your body** so you have tons of energy!

ating breakfast boosts your memory, helps you concentrate, boosts your mood, reduces your cholesterol levels and cuts your chances of developing diabetes or having a heart attack.

## DON'T FORGET THE KIDS

Kids who eat breakfast do better at school and are more likely to join in with sports and games. They tend to eat more healthily in general. So encourage them to fuel up before they go out. Also, try to encourage them to have a portion of fruit with their breakfast, such as banana or strawberries on cereals or porridge.

## START THE DAY WELL

For the ultimate power breakfast, grab a bowl of high-fibre cereal. Or try some wholemeal toast. Opt for low-fat milk or yoghurt – their calcium will keep your bones strong. Add some fruit – a glass of juice or some berries or a sliced banana with your cereal.

## BREAKFAST IDEAS

Try some of these combinations to start the day:

⭐ Wholegrain breakfast cereal with low-fat milk and fresh fruit
⭐ Slice of wholemeal toast with Marmite and some orange juice
⭐ Bowl of porridge (made with whole milk) with a sliced banana
⭐ Poached egg on wholemeal toast, plus half a grapefruit
⭐ Fruit smoothie made with a handful of blueberries, a small banana, a pot of whole-milk yoghurt and a little runny honey

## Myths & Facts

**FACT:** People who eat a healthy breakfast lose more weight than breakfast-skippers and eat fewer calories for their lunch and dinner.

## STILL WANT A FRY-UP?

See those greasy sausages and bacon? Just grill them and you'll get all the flavour and half the fat! The same goes for mushrooms. Don't fry the eggs, gently poach them instead. Never fry bread – lightly toast it, and if you want, lightly spread it with olive oil or sunflower margarine. If you follow these simple rules your 'fried breakfast' will actually be healthier than many cereals!

"I never miss breakfast – it's the best meal of the day."

IAN WRIGHT'S FITTER FAMILIES

# Lunch on the run

Lunch fuels you through your working day. **Never skip** this **important meal**, no matter how busy you are. Otherwise, you **risk an energy dip** mid-afternoon that could find you reaching for a **chocolate bar**.

**Myths & Facts**

**FACT:** The average person eats 230 sandwiches a year. That's a lot of bread and BLT – make sure you stick to healthy options.

**Y**our body needs nutrients at lunchtime to keep you going through the afternoon. Ideally, you should make this your main meal of the day with a lighter meal in the evening. But it isn't easy if you have to work over lunch or eat on the run.

## SANDWICHES

These are the most popular convenience food there is. Here's how you can make them the perfect lunch fuel too.

- Choose wholemeal or granary bread instead of white bread.
- Try wholemeal pitta bread or wraps for a change.
- Opt for lean fillings – chicken, turkey, ham, tuna or salmon.

- Vegetarian? Try hummus, peanut butter or cottage cheese instead of high-fat cheese and eggs.
- Stuff your sarnies with lots of salad. It counts towards your 5 a day.
- Swap mayo for low-fat salad cream.
- Spread with olive oil or sunflower margarine.

- If you're buying pre-packed sandwiches, choose ones labelled 'low fat' or 'healthy choice'.
- Steer clear of anything with coleslaw, mayo or bacon. They are too fatty and salty.

## LUNCH

Here's how you can fit healthy eating into your working day:

- ★ Prepare a healthy packed lunch and take it with you to work.
- ★ Buy a low-fat wholemeal sandwich, a yoghurt and some fruit instead of pie and chips at the pub.
- ★ Other healthy takeaway options include jacket potato with beans, a supermarket pasta or tuna salad, or fresh soup with a wholemeal roll.
- ★ If you eat in a canteen, choose jacket potatoes, grilled fish, salads and veggies – avoid rich sauces or anything fried.

### TOP TIPS FOR LUNCH OUT

Going out for lunch? Decide whether to have a starter or dessert but don't have both. Pass on the bread basket. For main courses, select a simple meat or fish dish with vegetables or salad. Steer clear of creamy sauces and anything described as crispy, breaded, *en croute*, battered or fried. Stick to mineral water or juice – alcohol slows down your brain power and piles on the calories. Order fresh fruit or sorbet for dessert. If you can't resist a richer dessert, you could share it with a colleague.

# Dinner time made easy

When you're back late from work or from picking up the kids, it's tempting to grab a ready meal or get a takeaway. But it **doesn't take much** to knock up a **healthy meal**. The key is to **plan ahead**. Stock up your fridge with healthy fresh food. That way, you can have **low-fat meals in minutes**.

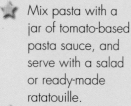

### MAKING READY MEALS HEALTHIER

Most ready meals are high in fat and salt. Try to have them just once a week. Here's how to make them healthier:

- Mix pasta with a jar of tomato-based pasta sauce, and serve with a salad or ready-made ratatouille.
- Beef up shepherd's pie by serving it with broccoli and carrots.
- Balance fish fingers and chips with heaps of green vegetables.

Cook meals at home as much as possible. Encourage your kids to help to prepare meals, choosing healthy, delicious foods – they're more likely to eat the meal if they've been involved with making it. Cooking can be great fun for kids and gives them a terrific sense of achievement. So get in the kitchen!

### SAME FOR ALL

The whole family will benefit from eating healthy meals. There's no need to prepare different meals for the kids. Most traditional family meals can be adapted easily to contain less fat.

### MORE FOR LATER

Save time by doubling up on a recipe – eat half and keep the rest in the fridge or freezer. All-in-one dishes such as soup, hot pots, Bolognese sauce, casseroles, pasta sauce and rice dishes are easy to make and freeze well. Streamline your cooking. Try:

- A tasty stir fry – prawns or chicken cooked in a wok with plenty of vegetables and served with rice
- A jacket potato with tuna, beans or cheese served with a big leafy salad
- A grilled skinless chicken or turkey breast served with lots of vegetables
- Wholemeal pasta mixed with pesto sauce or a tin of tuna or salmon
- A fish fillet, baked or grilled, served with lots of veggies and boiled rice
- Bolognese made with lean turkey or beef mince with spaghetti and vegetables

# "Make a big bowl of fruit salad and keep it in the fridge."

**Use less fat**
*Make healthy fish and chips by losing the fatty batter and pan-frying the fish in a little olive oil instead. Make oven-baked chips (see recipe) and you can still enjoy your favourite meal.*

## IAN'S EASY STAND-BYS

Deep-fried chips and burgers are unhealthy because of their fat content. Try these more healthy versions.

### Healthy home-made chips

Scrub a few potatoes, cut them in half lengthways then cut each half into six wedges. Place them in a baking tin and turn in a little olive oil until each piece is lightly coated. Bake at 200°C for 35 to 40 minutes until the potatoes are soft inside and golden brown on the outside.

### Healthy burgers

Mix together 175g lean mince, a small handful of dried breadcrumbs, half a chopped onion, 1 tbsp. chopped parsley, 2 tbsp. water and a little salt and pepper. Shape the mixture into four burgers, place on an oiled baking tray, brush with oil and bake at 200°C for 10 to15 minutes.

## TOP TIP

If your kids insist on snacking on junk food, try to limit them to one item a day. It won't do them any harm provided the rest of their diet is healthy and they're eating their 5 a day. Don't ban anything – it'll only make them want to eat it more. Instead, stock your larder and fridge with healthy choices and let them see you enjoying healthy snacks too.

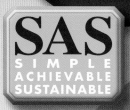

# SAS
SIMPLE
ACHIEVABLE
SUSTAINABLE

**Healthy snacks**
*We all love snacking, but make sure your snacks are mainly the healthy sort. Try plain popcorn for a crunchy treat.*

# Just a snack between meals

There's nothing wrong with snacking. It helps to **keep your energy up** between meals and, if you choose the right sort, a **snack can be good** for you too. Fresh fruit, for example, is packed with vitamins. And it **tastes delicious**!

**W**hat do you do when the hunger pangs strike? Reach for a chocolate bar or bag of crisps? They may fill a hole for a while but they're also loaded with bad fats, sugar and salt. Try swapping one of your usual snacks for something healthier.

## HEALTHY SNACKS – SWEET

Fruit cake or malt loaf • Fresh fruit, such as grapes, bananas or apples • Dried fruit • Low-fat fruit yoghurt • Smoothie (bought or home-made) • Cereal bars • Flavoured milk

## HEALTHY SNACKS – SAVOURY

Oatcakes and wholemeal crackers • Toast thinly spread with sunflower margarine • Rice cakes with peanut butter • Low-fat baked crisps • Unsalted nuts • Plain popcorn • Thin slice of cheese

| INSTEAD OF | EAT SOME |
|---|---|
| Crisps/salty packet snacks | Plain popcorn or Twiglets |
| Biscuits | Rice cakes with peanut butter or cheese |
| Croissant | Toast with Marmite |
| Cakes | Wholemeal fruit bun |
| Sweets | Dried apple rings, nuts |
| Chocolate bar | Cereal or breakfast bar |
| Cola | Water; low-fat milk or flavoured milk |

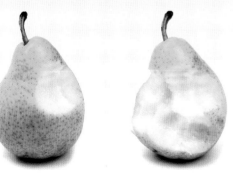
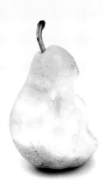

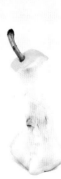

# Takeaways and eating out

Eating out is a treat, but unfortunately most of what's on the menu **isn't exactly healthy**. Takeaways and fast food meals can be **loaded** with **calories, fat, sugar** and **salt**. What you need is a **clever plan** of action.

**G**o for low-fat options, avoiding creamy sauces and deep-fried foods. If you don't know what's in a dish or how it's cooked, don't be afraid to ask. Refuse the 'supersize' or 'buy-one-get-one-free offers' and stick to standard portions. Don't over-order. Think about how much you would eat for a home-cooked meal and stick to similar amounts.

### EATING OUT TIPS

Choose main dishes that include plenty of vegetables or order extra vegetable side dishes (plain, not fried or smothered in butter or cream) with your main dish. If a dish comes with a sauce or dressing, ask for it to be served separately. Follow these eat-smart rules:

⭐ Choose grilled chicken rather than fried. It contains less fat and 160 fewer calories.

⭐ Don't lick your fingers when eating fried food – it can add an extra 100 calories!

⭐ Swap fries for salad or veg and save 260 calories.

**BAD FOOD**
Fast foods, such as hamburgers and pizzas are loaded with saturated fat and salt. A 2007 survey found that a pizza meal with garlic bread contained 9g of salt – more than an adult's entire daily maximum (6g).

## "Pass on the bread basket – it's tempting to overeat.

## TAKEAWAY HEAVEN

If you can't resist fish and chips, find a shop where they're crisp and not soggy. Chunky chips are better than skinny french fries because they soak up less fat. Fancy a burger? Just choose the smallest portion not the quarter-pounder. And if you must have a kebab, make it a shish kebab – grilled meat in pitta is a healthier option than a greasy doner kebab. Or try falafel. This is a tasty Middle Eastern patty made from chickpeas and served in pitta with salad.

## GOOD TAKEAWAY FOOD CHOICES

| | |
|---|---|
| **CHINESE** | Chicken chop suey; sweet and sour vegetables; vegetable spring roll |
| **INDIAN** | Chicken tikka; vegetable balti; plain rice; channa dahl |
| **PASTA** | Pasta with tomato/vegetable/seafood-based sauces; pasta filled with spinach |
| **PIZZA** | Thin-base pizza with vegetable toppings; salad with tomatoes and olives |
| **BURGERS** | Plain burger in a bun; salad without croutons or dressing |

## CHINESE

Chinese dishes are tasty but can be laden with salt, sugar and fat. Make sure you balance your menu with lots of vegetables, and go easy on the fried dishes.

⭐ Avoid 'battered', 'deep-fried' or 'crispy' options.
⭐ Order chop suey and stir-fried vegetables.
⭐ Choose boiled instead of fried rice.
⭐ Try lychees for a low-fat dessert.

## INDIAN

Indian dishes can be healthy provided you avoid oily sauces, ghee and cream.

⭐ Steer clear of kormas, masalas, rogan josh, biryanis and jaipuris because they are high in fat.
⭐ Choose dry-cooked dishes such as tandooris and ordinary tikkas.

### Thai choices

*Eating Thai? Give green and red curries a miss – they're usually swimming in oil. Go for stir-fried chicken, fish and veg.*

## PIZZA AND PASTA

Restaurant portions are usually huge – fine if you're a professional sportsperson, but most of us could end up overloading on calories. Stick to simple dishes!

⭐ Share a pizza – a whole one has 1,000 to 1,400 calories.
⭐ Opt for pizza with extra vegetable toppings.
⭐ Avoid meat toppings like pepperoni and ground beef – they're high in fat and salt.
⭐ Avoid pizzas with a stuffed crust.
⭐ Choose minestrone soup or a tomato salad for starters instead of garlic bread.
⭐ Choose simple tomato or vegetable sauces for pasta.

IAN WRIGHT'S FITTER FAMILIES

### TOP TIPS FOR HEALTHY EATING

Because takeaway foods are loaded with salt, they make you thirstier than usual. Don't be tempted to buy a fizzy drink – it won't quench your thirst and may make you put on more weight. Drink water instead.

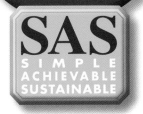

**SAS**
SIMPLE
ACHIEVABLE
SUSTAINABLE

# A little of what you fancy

Most of us enjoy a **tipple** now and then – one or two drinks a day can even be good for your heart. But **don't overdo it** – too much is **bad** for your health and can make you put on **weight**.

A glass (175ml) of red wine: 140 calories

Shot of whisky: 50 calories

## How much?

Men should drink no more than 3 or 4 units a day, and women 2 or 3 units. A unit is half a pint of beer or lager, or a single shot of spirits. A glass of wine is about 2 units.

A pint of beer: 140 calories

Myths & Facts

**FACT:** If you hold your glass in your hand at a party, you will drink more quickly than if you put it down on a nearby table.

A glass (125ml) of Buck's fizz: 75 calories

"There are some truly great alternatives when it comes to non-alcoholic drinks."

Next time you fancy a party drink but without the hangover risk, try this refreshing non-alcoholic cocktail.

### GINGER SPLICE

3 carrots
1/2 small fennel bulb
1 large celery stick
root ginger

Place the ingredients in a blender or juicer and blitz. Serve in a chilled glass over crushed ice.

## Myths & Facts

**MYTH:** It's a myth that you can burn fat from specific regions of your body. When you exercise, you burn fat from all areas of your body, not just the part involved in the exercise.

# Action stations!

It's time to get off the sofa and **get moving!** In this section you'll find lots of ideas for **increasing your activity** and **burning off calories.** Try walking, hiking, cycling, running or swimming – they're all great ways of **boosting your fitness**. I've put together a four-week plan for each activity to **help get you started.**

# On your feet

**Walking** is the **easiest** and cheapest exercise of all. You've been doing it all your **life**. Whether it's for exercise, a **stroll** or to walk the dog, there are **lots of benefits** to be gained.

## TOP WALKING TIPS

- Relax your shoulders to improve posture. Keep them down but not back.
- Hold your arms relaxed, close to your sides. Avoid swinging them across your body.
- Walk tall, not tensed and hunched. Look forwards not down.
- Walk heel to toe and keep a comfortable stride length.
- Keep your hips, knees and feet in a straight line. Your feet should point directly forwards.

Aim to walk at least 30 minutes a day at least five days a week. If this is too much, you can build up to this. You can split the walking into two or three shorter sessions. But it's important that you do it regularly, on most days of the week. The more you do, the more you benefit.

## WHY IT'S GOOD FOR YOU

Walking burns fat if you keep a good pace, pump your arms and walk on an incline whenever possible. It strengthens your heart and tones your leg muscles if you do it regularly.

## SPEED CHECK

You should be walking faster than a stroll and be slightly breathless. You should be able to talk in short sentences. Up your speed when you no longer feel challenged; reduce it if you feel uncomfortable.

## WHAT TO WEAR

When you take up walking as a serious form of exercise, good shoes are a must. Invest in comfortable walking shoes if you don't have any. They should feel roomy around the toes, provide good heel cushioning and be comfortable and light. In warm weather, wear light, loose clothing. In cold weather, wear layers so that you can remove some of the outer ones as you get hotter.

"Walking is one of the simplest ways of getting fit."

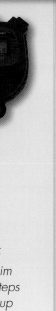

**Keeping count**
*Pedometers are
a good way of
keeping track of
your exercise. Aim
to do 10,000 steps
a day but build up
gradually. Every step
counts, even just
walking around at
home or work.*

## SAS
### SIMPLE
### ACHIEVABLE
### SUSTAINABLE

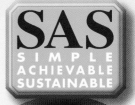

### WALKING
### IS GOOD FOR YOU
If you walk for 45 minutes
four times a week you could lose
8 kilos of fat over a year.

A study at Harvard University
found that people who walked
5 to 10 miles a week had a
25% lower risk of having
heart disease.

IAN WRIGHT'S FITTER FAMILIES

# Build up gradually

When you take up walking, start at a **comfortable pace** and increase slowly. Doing too much **too fast** can lead to **injuries** and set you back instead of move you forwards.

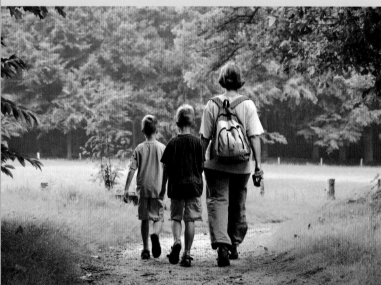

If you can do only a five-minute walk, then start by walking just five minutes two or three days per week, maybe as slowly as 1mph. If you already walk occasionally but want to make it a habit, walk for at least ten minutes perhaps at 2 or 3mph, three days per week.

## BUILD UP GRADUALLY

Every one to two weeks, bump up your frequency a notch by adding one more day per week. In a month, you should be walking four or five days per week, even if you don't increase how fast or how long you walk. When you're ready to make a second increase, choose either to walk the same distance faster or walk a few minutes longer at your usual pace.

## FOUR-WEEK WALKING PROGRAMME

Adjust your pace and the length of your walk as necessary. You may find you're walking faster and longer – and reaping more health benefits – without knowing it. Aim to walk for 30 minutes or more at least five times a week. Build up gradually with this four-week programme (below). Don't forget: SAS! If this is too much too soon for you, take it at a slower pace.

| | No. of workouts per week | Warm-up (walk slowly) | Main walk (walk briskly) | Cool-down (walk slowly) | Total exercise time |
|---|---|---|---|---|---|
| **WEEK 1** | 3 | 5 minutes | 5 minutes | 5 minutes | 15 minutes |
| **WEEK 2** | 3–4 | 5 minutes | 10 minutes | 5 minutes | 20 minutes |
| **WEEK 3** | 4–5 | 5 minutes | 15 minutes | 5 minutes | 25 minutes |
| **WEEK 4** | 5 | 5 minutes | 20 minutes | 5 minutes | 30 minutes |

# "Make walking a daily habit."

## TOP TIPS

Avoid injury by warming up with some shoulder rolls and knee raises. Do some simple calf and thigh stretches (see pages 150–151). Hold a stretch for eight to ten seconds. Repeat after your workout.

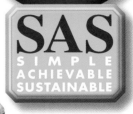

## SAS

**SIMPLE
ACHIEVABLE
SUSTAINABLE**

**Daily walk**
*Use every opportunity to walk each day
– take the kids to school on foot.*

## Myths & Facts

**FACT:** The average person travels 307km (192 miles) a year on foot – less than 3% of their overall distance travelled.

# Take a hike!

Any kind of walking is a **brilliant** way of getting fit but hiking on trails and tracks or up a hill is **much more fun** than pounding the pavements. It also works your legs a bit harder so you burn **more calories**.

The varying terrain improves your fitness more quickly than walking on the flat. Like walking, hiking is really good for your heart, lungs and leg muscles. If you walk uphill, it burns around 500 calories an hour. It strengthens your bones even more than walking on the flat but puts less stress on the joints than running. Exercising in the great outdoors reduces stress and boosts your mood.

## WHAT TO WEAR
Even if you only plan weekend walking every so often, wearing the right gear is a must. Make sure you're kitted out with the right gear before you set out.

- Take a waterproof/windproof jacket that lets out water vapour. It should have a large hood and be big enough to wear over several layers of clothing.
- Wear several thin layers – modern wicking fabrics such as Cool-Max are good for keeping cool.
- In hot weather, wear loose, lightweight clothing that is sweat permeable and pale coloured.
- Wear a hat – to prevent heat loss in winter, and to protect your head from the sun in summer.
- Walking boots or shoes with moulded grip-giving soles are a must if the ground is at all hilly or rough. Fitting should be snug but not over-tight.

## WHERE TO GO
www.go4awalk.com has maps you can print and info on walking in the UK. www.footpath-holidays.com has details of guided and non-guided holidays in the UK.

### Out in the country
*Hiking is a great way of exploring the countryside. Don't forget to take sensible clothing and a rucksack.*

### Correctly fitting boots
*The sides of your boots should support your ankle. The toe and heel should have strengthening to give extra protection.*

# Made it!

Hiking is the closest activity to **perfect exercise**, the most sustainable means of transport and Britain's most **popular** outdoor recreation by far. Whether you are planning a hiking holiday or just want to get fit, **build up gradually**.

**C**hoose a gentle route to begin with, then select more hilly routes or rougher terrain as you get fitter. If you are hiking longer than one hour, take a short break about every 30 minutes or whenever you feel you need a rest.

## WHAT TO TAKE WITH YOU

Take some food and drink, even if the walk includes a pub or café break. Be prepared for changing weather and any unfortunate accidents. Here's a list of must-haves.

 Something in which to carry first-aid equipment, a map and compass, an extra sweater and your supplies.

A drink – obey your thirst and drink little and often.

Make use of natural supplies whenever possible.

Food – for a day trip take a couple of sandwiches per person, peanuts, some dried fruit, a cereal bar, a bar of chocolate and (ideally) 2 litres of water.

Sunscreen – use high protection sunscreen (minimum SPF 15) on all exposed areas, not forgetting under your chin, your lips and your ears. In high temperatures, keep out of the sun during the hottest part of the day.

## A SIXTEEN-WEEK WALKING PROGRAMME

Whether you are planning a hiking holiday or just want to get fit, build up gradually with this 16-week programme. Aim to complete one hike a week to start with, say at the weekends, then add another as you get fitter.

"Make sure you have plenty of fresh water with you on any hike."

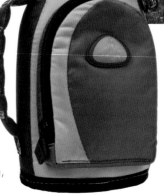

Useful item
*A rucksack is the best thing for taking supplies and equipment. It is easier to carry weight on your back than in one hand and then the other.*

**HIKING**
If you don't want to walk on your own, try a group walk. There are different levels of difficulty. Many are suitable for families. See www.ramblers.org.uk/info/localgroups.

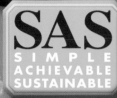

SAS
SIMPLE
ACHIEVABLE
SUSTAINABLE

| | No. of hikes per week | Warm-up (walk slowly) | Main hike (walk briskly) | Cool-down (walk slowly) | Total exercise time |
|---|---|---|---|---|---|
| **WEEKS 1–4** | 1–2 | 5 minutes | 45 mins – 1 hour | 5 minutes | 55 mins – 1 hr 10 mins |
| **WEEKS 5–8** | 1–2 | 5 minutes | 1 – 1½ hours | 5 minutes | 1 hr 10 mins – 1 hr 40 mins |
| **WEEKS 9–12** | 1–2 | 5 minutes | 1½ – 2 hours | 5 minutes | 1 hr 40 mins – 2 hr 10 mins |
| **WEEKS 13–16** | 1–2 | 5 minutes | 2 – 2½ hours | 5 minutes | 2 hr 10 mins – 2 hr 40 mins |

# Come along for the ride

**Cycling** is a great form of exercise as well as being a cheap and **pollution-free** means of getting about. Cycle to and from work or the shops and you'll be **integrating** exercise into your daily activities.

Cycling improves your heart and lungs and is a brilliant way to burn calories (around 450 calories per hour). It tones the muscles in your thighs, buttocks and lower legs and strengthens the lower back and stomach muscles.

## ALONG FOR THE RIDE

It's important to position yourself correctly on the bike. Feeling comfortable will help ensure that you don't put unnecessary strain on any part of your body.

- Saddle height – your legs should be extended in the downward phase of the cycling action.
- Keep your neck and shoulders relaxed.
- Your arms should be slightly bent at the elbows.
- Keep a firm but relaxed grip on the handles.
- Hold your stomach muscles tight – this will help to stabilise you.

## SAFETY FIRST

Always wear a well fitting helmet. Carry a basic toolkit and a spare inner tube. Wear bright colours and fluorescent strips and use lights in poor visibility. And follow the Highway Code.

## WHAT TO WEAR

A tracksuit, a cotton or polyester top and a pair of trainers are all you need. In cold weather, wear several thin layers under a cycling jersey or sweat top.

## TAKE IT STEADY

If you've not ridden a bike for some time, then it's worth taking things slowly at first. Don't rush, expecting instant results. Even if you are fit from being active in other sports, cycling does use muscles in a different way from, say, running, so you'll need to allow a bit of time for your body to adjust and get used to the new demands. Take things at a pace you're comfortable with and build up slowly in the SAS style.

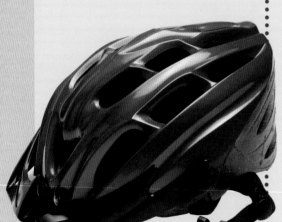

**Safety first**
*Make sure your helmet fits snugly. It should sit squarely on your head so it sits just above your eyebrows and is not tilted back or tipped forwards.*

IAN WRIGHT'S FITTER FAMILIES

"Get cycling in the fresh air on- or off-road, alone or with the whole family."

Myths & Facts

**FACT:** You can cycle four times faster than you can walk using the same amount of energy. You can cycle 1,037km (644 miles) on the energy equivalent of 1 litre of petrol.

# Pace yourself

If you rode a **bike** as a child it will come back to you quite **quickly**. Start in traffic-free areas and on **level ground** to build up your confidence. Introduce your **bottom** to the saddle slowly!

**B**egin with a maximum of 30 minutes to break yourself in gently. Then gradually build up the length of time you spend in the saddle. If you have knee problems, make sure the seat is high enough and the tension is low – keep in a low gear. If you have back problems, avoid bending forwards in the saddle.

### PEDAL RIGHT

Keep the ball of your foot on the pedal. A fairly brisk pedalling cadence is the most efficient – you can keep a steady speed without getting too tired. Aim for between 75 and 100 revolutions per minute (rpm). To find your rpm, count the revolutions in ten seconds then multiply by six. Use your gears to maintain the cadence.

### JOIN A CLUB

It is easier and more fun to cycle with other people. Ask bike shops for details of local cycling clubs. Some may offer fun days out in the country or competitions.

### FOUR-WEEK CYCLING PROGRAMME

Build up gradually starting with rides on the flat. Then pick more hilly routes as your fitness improves. It pays to do a little planning before you set off, so check your route on a map first.

**Stopping cramp**
*If you get foot cramps, check your laces aren't too tight, and avoid gripping with your toes.*

**CYCLING TOP TIPS**
Padded cycling gloves will keep your hands warm, protect them from blisters and absorb vibrations from the road.

**SAS**
SIMPLE
ACHIEVABLE
SUSTAINABLE

| | No. of rides per week | Warm-up (cycle slowly) | Main ride | Cool-down (cycle slowly) | Total workout time |
|---|---|---|---|---|---|
| **WEEK 1** | 3 | 5 minutes | 15 minutes | 5 minutes | 25 minutes |
| **WEEK 2** | 4–5 | 5 minutes | 20 minutes | 5 minutes | 30 minutes |
| **WEEK 3** | 4–5 | 5 minutes | 25 minutes | 5 minutes | 35 minutes |
| **WEEK 4** | 5 | 5 minutes | 30 minutes | 5 minutes | 40 minutes |

# Hit the ground running

Running is one of the **simplest** ways to get fit. You don't need to be sporty or very well co-ordinated and you can do it **where** and **when you like**. There is no special equipment, and no membership fee to pay.

**R**unning outdoors can be really exhilarating. It burns more calories than most other forms of aerobic exercise (around 100 calories per mile), so will whittle away those love handles fast!

## RUNNING THE RIGHT WAY

Running with good form will make it feel easier and help to prevent injuries. Poor technique can cause pain in the lower back and hips. Here's how to run:

⭐ Relax your shoulders and run upright. Keep your back straight and tall.
⭐ Keep your feet close to the ground and take care not to bounce as you run.
⭐ Let your arms swing backwards and forwards naturally. Keep your hands loose and tension-free.

## HOW TO GET STARTED

Make sure that you feel confident with fast walking first – you should be able to walk for 30 minutes easily. Begin with interval running, when you run for short periods then walk fast until you recover. Gradually make the running intervals longer and build up the length of your workout.

## GETTING STITCHES

Stitches are common in beginners because the abdomen is not used to all that jostling. Breathe deeply to stretch out the diaphragm (just below your lungs). Stitches usually go away as you get fitter. Also, try to avoid eating in the hour before you run.

## WHAT TO WEAR

⭐ Comfortable jogging trousers or shorts
⭐ A good pair of running shoes rather than all-round trainers
⭐ A supportive bra and a T-shirt or sweat top

**Myths & Facts**

**FACT:** You can reduce your risk of stroke by 63% if you run regularly for 20 to 40 minutes three to five times a week.

### FEELING OUT OF BREATH

You should just about be able to hold a conversation while you run. If you feel out of breath, slow down and take a walking break. Breathe from deep down in your belly. Most of that out-of-breath feeling diminishes as you get fitter.

# "Having a running partner can make all the difference and really spur you on."

# Running for fun

You can **run anywhere** that's safe and enjoyable. Choose **scenic** routes that are well lit and not congested with traffic. Run on **smooth** grass or trails, rather than roads, whenever you can to save your joints.

**B**efore you start running, do five minutes' brisk walking. This prepares your body and helps to avoid injury. After your run, walk slowly for five minutes then do some stretches for your calves and thighs (see pages 150–151).

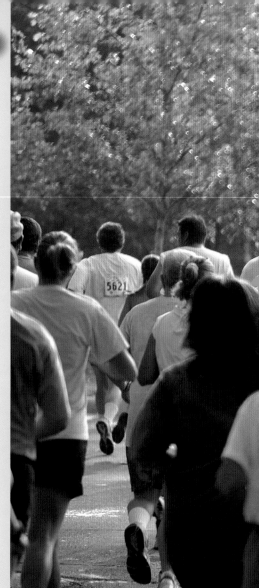

**Running indoors**
*With no wind, running on a treadmill is slightly easier than running outside.*

### TAKING IT SLOWLY

To start with, try to find a pace that's faster than a walk. As you get fitter you can up your pace. Remember there's no right or wrong here. The important thing is to feel that you're challenging yourself a little but not gasping for breath.

### JOIN OTHER PEOPLE

Visit www.runnersweb.co.uk for details of clubs in your area, charity runs and, when you're feeling up to them, marathons. Organised runs are fun if you don't overdo it.

### FOUR-WEEK RUNNING PROGRAMME

This beginner's programme alternates running with walking breaks. This allows you to build from walking to running for almost 20 minutes within four weeks. Allow at least a day between runs when you begin.

IAN WRIGHT'S FITTER FAMILIES

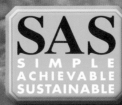

**SIMPLE ACHIEVABLE SUSTAINABLE**

**CHARITY RUN**
You can enter a fun run soon after taking up running. Don't worry if you need to walk some of the way – lots of people do. Fun runs are usually held as a sideshow to a bigger race. Distances start at one mile, and few are longer than two or three. For details of what's on in your area and how to enter, log on to www. runnersworld.co.uk.

|  | No. of workouts per week | Warm-up | Workout | Cool-down | Total workout time |
|---|---|---|---|---|---|
| **WEEK 1** | 3 | Walk for 5 minutes | Run 30 seconds, walk 1 minute. Repeat 10 times | Walk slowly 3 minutes, stretch 2 minutes | 25 minutes |
| **WEEK 2** | 3–4 | Walk for 5 minutes | Run 1 minute, walk 1 minute. Repeat 10 times | Walk slowly 3 minutes, stretch 2 minutes | 30 minutes |
| **WEEK 3** | 3–4 | Walk for 5 minutes | Run 2 minutes, walk 1 minute. Repeat 7 times | Walk slowly 3 minutes, stretch 2 minutes | 31 minutes |
| **WEEK 4** | 3–4 | Walk for 5 minutes | Run 3 minutes, walk 1 minute. Repeat 5 times | Walk slowly 3 minutes, stretch 2 minutes | 30 minutes |

**TOP TIPS**

Aim to keep your body 'long' and stretched out in the water.

Make every stroke count. Use as few strokes as possible to swim each length.

# Sink or swim

Swimming is **relaxing** and **simple**. It's a great way to get fit and have **fun**. Most towns have a pool so you can fit a swim into your working day or enjoy a **family swim** at weekends.

Swimming is thought to be one of the best workouts you can give your body because it works almost all of your major muscle groups at the same time. Since you're floating in the water and not in contact with any hard surfaces, there's less pressure on your joints and bones. You're a lot less likely to suffer certain kinds of injuries than with other sports.

## IMPROVING YOUR STROKE

How fast or how far you swim is not as important as the amount of time you spend swimming. Doing it more often and for longer periods of time provides better exercise. Here are some easy tips on improving your front crawl.

- Turn your head to the side to breathe in, rather than lifting your head out of the water.
- Breathe out while under water as you pull through from mid-stroke to the end of the stroke.
- Reach directly in front of you. Keep your hand slightly cupped as you pull through the stroke.
- Kick from your hip, using your entire leg not just the part below your knee.

## TIPS FOR BEGINNERS

If swimming a length is too far to start with, swim widths, gradually building up the number until you can swim the distance for a length. Once you can swim a length you can gradually build up the number of lengths you swim at each session and then start to swim continuously for a set time. Remember: SAS!

## EQUIPMENT

If you are new to swimming, use a float to provide buoyancy. Hold it in front of you with both hands as you kick your legs.

> "Pretend you're a fish, a dolphin, a shark ..."

# In the swim

**Water** can feel relaxing, but if you are trying to improve your fitness you will need to **push yourself a little**. You should not be able to talk comfortably – just one-word answers if **pushed**!

There are many ways to push yourself and get better as a swimmer. If you're into speed, you can race the clock and see how long it takes you to do a certain number of lengths. If you're into endurance, you can slow down and see how many lengths you can do before you have to rest.

### TAKING IT SLOWLY

Most public pools have lanes for different speeds and levels. You can work at your own pace and use any stroke style. If you need to work on your stroke technique, ask about group lessons or sign up for one-to-one instruction.

### HOW TO BREATHE

Practise breathing using a float. Put one arm on the float, holding it close to your body, and use the other arm to pull through the stroke. As you breathe in, turn your head away from the float. Breathe out into the water.

### FOUR-WEEK SWIMMING PROGRAMME

The warm-up should feel fairly easy, so focus on your technique. Change the strokes you are doing from time to time – alternate between front crawl and back crawl or front crawl and breaststroke. Take a rest if you are too tired.

|  | No. of workouts per week | Warm-up (Use a variety of strokes) | Workout | Cool-down (Use a variety of strokes) | Total workout time |
|---|---|---|---|---|---|
| **WEEK 1** | 2 | 4 lengths at a comfortable pace | Swim for 15 minutes: 1 length fast, 1 length recovery | 6 lengths at a comfortable pace | 25 minutes |
| **WEEK 2** | 3 | 4 lengths at a comfortable pace | Swim for 20 minutes: 1 length fast, 1 length recovery | 6 lengths at a comfortable pace | 30 minutes |
| **WEEK 3** | 3–4 | 6 lengths at a comfortable pace | Swim for 25 minutes: 2 lengths fast, 1 length recovery | 6 lengths at a comfortable paces | 35 minutes |
| **WEEK 4** | 3–4 | 6 lengths at a comfortable pace | Swim for 30 minutes: 2 lengths fast, 1 lengths recovery | 6 lengths at a comfortable paces | 40 minutes |

IAN WRIGHT'S FITTER FAMILIES

Myths
&
Facts

**FACT:** An hour of vigorous swimming will burn up to 650 calories. It burns off more calories than walking or cycling.

# Fun for

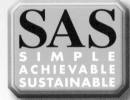

**LUCKY DIP!**
Write some enjoyable activities, such as dancing, football and swimming, on pieces of paper and put these in a jar. Take it in turns to pick a different activity to do every day or every week. By varying your activities, you are less likely to get bored.

**Nothing extra**
*You don't need any equipment to get fit. Comfy clothes and a bit of space is all that's needed. Use your imagination and let the kids take you for a ride!*

# all the family

It's important for everyone in your family to **keep active**. You don't need to be super-competitive or brilliant at sports to be active. Try some of the **fun games** described in the next section. They're suitable for all ages and you'll **all have fun** getting fit together.

*Myths & Facts*

**FACT:** In a study by University College London, only 6% of parents with overweight or obese children described their child as overweight.

# "You could have at least an hour's fun here."

## EQUIPMENT

⭐ 5 balls (not too bouncy) or bean bags and something to mark out a target (eg. chalk, sticks, string)

## WHERE

⭐ You need a bit of space outside for this game. Maybe you could play it in your local park. Just make sure you've got enough room to throw the balls without hitting anyone!

# Target practice

## ACTIVITY

Mark out a circular target zone about 3–5 metres from a throwing line. Have a bronze, silver and gold section. Make the gold the smallest and most difficult circle but not impossible. Gold gives you 10 points, silver 5 points and bronze 2 points.

Start by standing behind the line and throwing the ball towards the target. Have five throws each and see who wins.

OK, that was easy. Now turn around and face backwards and try five throws again. Who is winning now?

OK, OK, still too easy? Then try lying flat on your back, bend your knees and have your feet flat on the ground. Now sit up and throw. You must lie down again between each throw. This is a great one to give you a strong stomach.

Still easy? OK, try standing up with your back to the target and throwing the ball through your legs. Who is the winner?

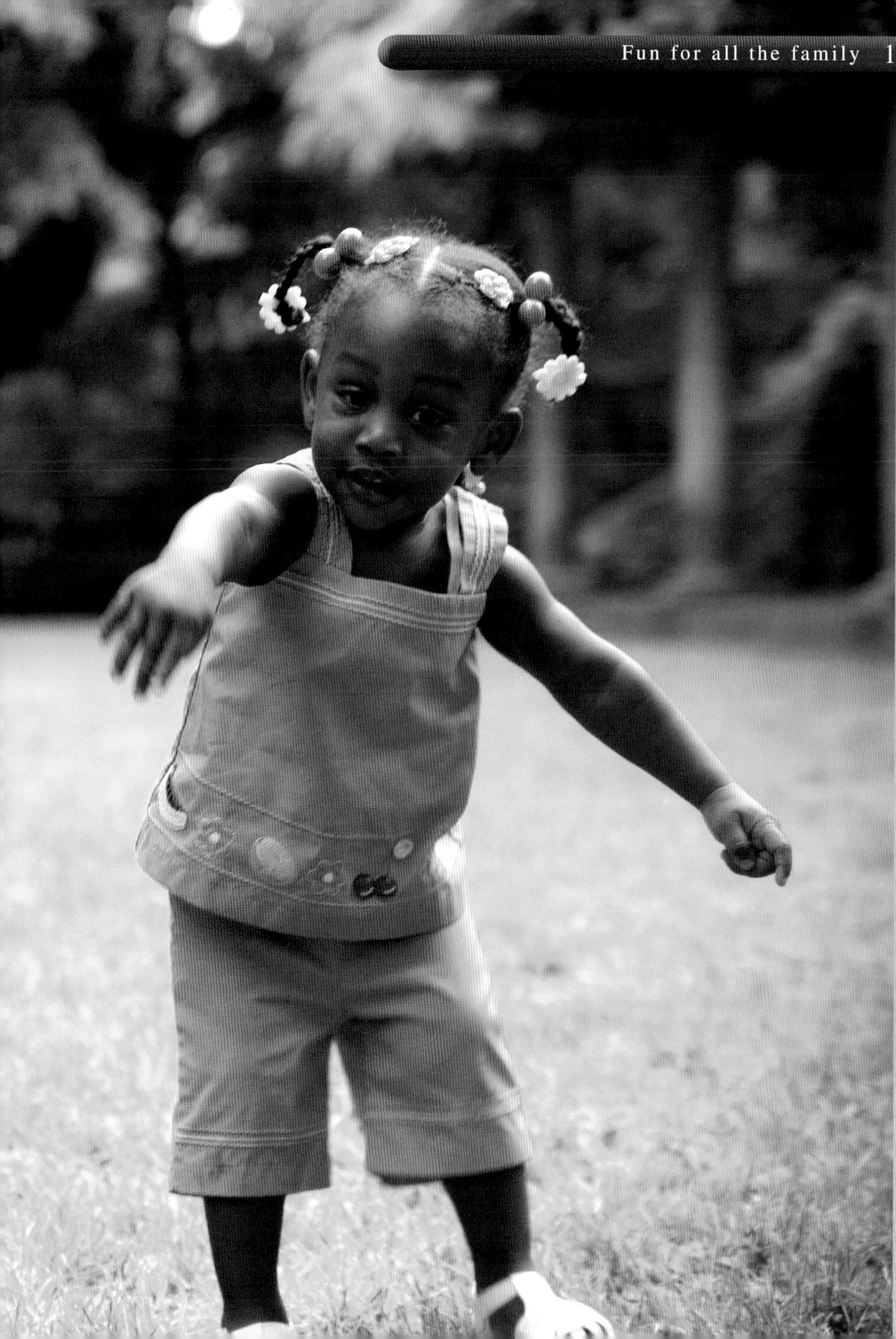

# Topsy turvy

## EQUIPMENT
⭐ Coloured pieces of card or plastic plates with two different coloured or shaped faces and plain backs. You can make your own by marking one side with a bold star or painting it a different colour.

## WHERE
⭐ Best played in an open space outside

## ACTIVITY

Place the cards all over the ground, with the two different colours or shapes facing upwards. Divide yourself into two teams, each choosing a different colour or shape.

Stand in opposite corners and on the command of 'Go', start to turn the cards so that your team's colour is facing up and the other team's colour is facing down. The aim is for each team (or person) to turn over as many of the cards as possible to their colour. The other team will be turning them back so you'll have to be quick! Play for three or four minutes and then the person that shouted 'Go' shouts 'Stop'. See who has the most of their colour facing upwards.

Replay the game changing colours.

This game can be really tiring so you should feel very out of breath!

# "This is a great family game to play all year round. Sure to get you ready for dinner!"

# Catch and aim

## EQUIPMENT
⭐ One ball, any type

## WHERE
⭐ Best played outside, maybe in the local park

## ACTIVITY

One of you throws the ball up as high as they can and shouts someone's name. That person must catch the ball while the rest of you run away. When they catch the ball they shout, 'Stop!' and you must all stop. The catcher can then take three steps and throw the ball to try to hit one of the group. If they manage it, the hit person then throws the ball up and everything starts again.

If you want to make this even more fun, kick the ball as high as you can – but it must go straight up in the air, not forwards.

# Pass and swap

### ACTIVITY

To start with, stand in pairs facing each other, about five or six good steps apart. You can move further apart as you become better at this game!

Start by passing the ball backwards and forwards to each other using a chest pass, then every sixth pass both of you shout, 'Swap!' and change places. When you have got this, try passing faster and change every four passes.

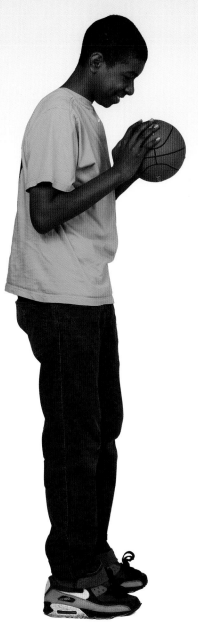

If you drop the ball during this game, you have to sit on the ground and stand up three times, as quickly as you can. This will help to give you really strong legs.

Change the way you pass the ball: use a bounce pass, left-hand throw and left-hand catch, overhead pass, through-the-legs-backwards pass, or a jump and pass.

Now try something a bit tougher! Every time you pass the ball, spin round before the ball comes back to you.

Finally, try touching the ground with your hand before the next pass comes.

Don't forget to shout, 'Swap!' and change places.

| EQUIPMENT |
| :--- |
| ⭐ A ball (football-sized) |

| WHERE |
| :--- |
| ⭐ Outside |

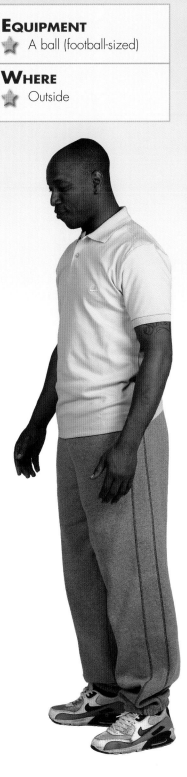

## Myths & Facts

**FACT:** The average couch potato's heart beats 70–75 times per minute. An active person's heart can pump the same amount of blood in only 50 beats.

# Twist, turn and travel

## ACTIVITY

Split into two teams and make two lines with the equipment. Place a skipping rope first, then a hurdle, then a hoop and finally a garden chair. Have a few metres between each item.

The first person runs out and does 15 skips, then runs to the hurdle and jumps forwards and backwards over it 10 times.

Next, they jump in and out of the hoop 10 times. Then they run around the garden chair and run back to their team. Then the next person does the same. Each team member should complete the obstacle course at least three or four times. The team to finish first is the winner.

## EQUIPMENT
⭐ 2 skipping ropes, 2 hoops, 2 hurdles (or other small objects to jump over), 2 garden chairs

## WHERE
⭐ Best played outside in lots of space

# Fruit salad

## ACTIVITY

Everyone sits in a circle. One person (person A) goes around the circle giving each person the name of a fruit. The number of fruits used depends on the number of people playing, but usually three or four different fruits are used. More than one person can have the same fruit name.

Person A calls out the name of one of the fruits. Everyone with that fruit name runs around the outside of the circle in a clockwise direction back to their space and sits down.

## OTHER RULES

This game can be made into a race, so that the last person back to their space is out or loses a life. Person A can call out more than one fruit at a time.

If person A calls out, 'Fruit salad!' everyone runs around the circle at the same time. If person A calls out, 'Smoothie!' the people running must spin around once and then carry on running.

## EQUIPMENT
⭐ None

## WHERE
⭐ Somewhere with enough room to run around

### SAFETY TIPS
Make sure that everyone runs in the same direction in order to avoid accidents! Those who are not running must keep their hands inside the circle, so that they don't trip the people who are running.

# Stepping stones

## EQUIPMENT

⭐ At least 2 hoops (4 is better); a pile of junk items or clothes

## WHERE

⭐ You need space for this game – maybe in the park

## ACTIVITY

Start off doing this activity in pairs. You need two hoops per pair. Each pair has to get from the start to the finishing line by jumping from hoop to hoop, both at the same time without stepping out of the hoops. Jump into one hoop then reach back for the other and place it in front of you. Use different-sized hoops to make things more interesting.

Once you have mastered this, the pairs could race each other. If anyone steps or falls out of a hoop the pair must go back to the beginning and start again.

Make this more difficult but still have great fun by all going together using three or four hoops. For this, you will need to work together to work out who goes when – you probably won't all fit in one hoop.

Try the game again, but carrying the junk or clothes. It's more difficult – and more fun – if you use balls or big items. You could time each other and add a ten-second penalty for every item dropped.

# Cats and mice

## ACTIVITY

Lay the hoops all over the ground several metres apart. If there are four of you, put out at least eight hoops to begin with. One person needs to be the first cat, and their job is to try to catch the mice. The mice run around, in and out of the areas between the hoops but not in them. The cat counts to ten then tries to catch the mice before they jump into a hoop, where they are safe. If a mouse is caught, they become a cat. Keep going until all the mice have been caught.

### Make it tougher

*Try taking away one or two hoops so that there aren't enough hoops for all the mice.*

## EQUIPMENT

⭐ Hoops or anything that can make smallish circles

## WHERE

⭐ Somewhere with plenty of space

"Parents, why not challenge your kids to this game?"

# Duck, duck, goose

**EQUIPMENT**
⭐ Hoops for forfeits

**WHERE**
⭐ Outside

## ACTIVITY

Sit down in a circle facing each other. One person is 'It' and walks around the circle. As they walk around, they tap people's heads and say whether they are the goose or a duck.

Once someone is the goose they get up and try to chase It around the circle of ducks. The goose's aim is to tag It before he or she is able to sit down in the goose's spot. If the goose is not able to do this, they become It for the next round and the play continues. If the goose does tag It, It has to do a forfeit then sit in the centre of the circle of ducks. Then the goose becomes It for the next round. The person in the middle can't leave until another It is tagged and they are replaced.

**Forfeits!**
*Use your imagination to think of an active forfeit. How about five star jumps, hula-hooping for ten seconds, three forward rolls or a silly dance?*

**SAFETY TIPS**
Remember to tag each other gently rather than with a hard slap! Make sure you don't lean back when sitting in the circle, and keep your hands inside the circle so that they don't trip or harm other people (or yourself).

Sssssh!
*Move quickly, but make sure
the bear can't hear you – you
don't want to get caught!*

# Look out bear!

## ACTIVITY

Everybody sits in a circle, with one person in the middle covering their eyes. This person is the bear. The bear has the ball in front of them. The ball is the bear's honey.

One person from the circle tiptoes to the honey and 'steals' it. Everyone else in the circle shouts, 'Look out bear!' and the bear chases the honey-stealer around the circle back to their space. (If the bear hears the honey-stealer, then he or she can catch the thief red-handed.) The bear's aim is to tag the honey-stealer and get back the honey. If the bear catches the honey-stealer, then the honey-stealer becomes the bear. If the honey-stealer escapes, then the bear returns to the middle and plays again until they catch someone.

There's no winner in this game but you'll have a lot of fun stealing the bear's honey!

| EQUIPMENT | |
|---|---|
| ⭐ | Soft ball or bean bag |

| WHERE | |
|---|---|
| ⭐ | Anywhere with space |

Myths
**FACT:** Research has shown that 95% of children who enjoy exercise as a child continue this into adulthood. So make sure it's fun!
Facts

# What's the time, Mr Wolf?

| EQUIPMENT |
|---|
| ⭐ None |

| WHERE |
|---|
| ⭐ Anywhere with space |

## ACTIVITY

One player is the wolf and stands with their back to the others, at least 5 metres away. Everyone starts to move towards the wolf, the aim being to get close enough to touch him or her and be wolf next. They call out, 'What's the time, Mr Wolf?' and the wolf shouts out a time, for example 10 o'clock. The wolf can turn round at any time. Everyone must then stay still, because if the wolf sees someone move, that person must return to the start.

The wolf then turns away again. The others continue to move forwards asking, 'What's the time, Mr Wolf?' and he says another time. When the wolf thinks the group are close enough to be caught, he calls out, 'Dinner time!' and chases them. Everyone must try to run back to the start line before the wolf catches them. The wolf has to be careful that he doesn't wait too long before dinner time and allows someone to get close enough to touch him.

### SAFETY TIPS
You'll all be running as fast as possible to escape Mr Wolf, but be careful! Always make sure you have your own space when running and turning.

"Playing should always be fun – even if you fall on your bum!"

# Chain tag

| EQUIPMENT |
| --- |
| ⭐ None |

| WHERE |
| --- |
| ⭐ Anywhere with lots of space |

## ACTIVITY

To start, one person is chosen as 'It' and has to try to tag another player. Everyone has to avoid being tagged so you'll all need to move as fast as you can. Once you have been tagged, you join hands with It and the two of you have to try to tag another player. That player then joins hands with you, forming a chain, and you continue to try to tag other players. If the chain becomes too long, you can split into smaller tag teams. The last person to be tagged is the winner and begins the next game as It.

*Spread the game over a bigger distance to get people running and out of breath when the wolf's back is turned!*

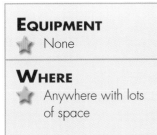

# Simon says

**EQUIPMENT**
 None

**WHERE**
⭐ Anywhere with space

### SAFETY TIPS
Just be aware of space constraints, so that you don't bump into each other or accidentally hit each other.

### ACTIVITY
One person is chosen to be Simon. Everyone else stands in a straight line. Simon gives instructions such as, 'Simon says, touch your ears,' and then everyone must follow the instruction. It can be anything like 'touch your toes', 'jump ten times on one foot' or 'spin around'. But if Simon gives the instruction without saying, 'Simon says,' first, then no one should do the action – anyone who does, loses a life or is out and has to sit down. The last person left standing can then be Simon.

### OTHER RULES
Simon can change the pace at which instructions are given. The faster the instructions are given, the more difficult it is for everyone.

# In and out the pond

**EQUIPMENT**
⭐ None

**WHERE**
⭐ Anywhere

### ACTIVITY
One person is the instructor. Everyone else stands along a line. When the instructor shouts, 'In the pond,' everyone jumps forwards over the line. When the instructor shouts, 'Out the pond,' they jump back. The instructor repeats both commands until people start getting them wrong.

If a person jumps 'in the pond' when the command is 'out the pond', that person is out. The instructor keeps going until there is only one person left – the winner!

### OTHER RULES
The instructor can increase the speed of the commands to make it trickier for everyone else!

# Groovy greetings

**EQUIPMENT**
⭐ None

**WHERE**
⭐ Anywhere

### ACTIVITY
Everyone walks, jumps, jogs, hops or skips around and shakes the hand of as many people as possible in two minutes.

### OTHER RULES
Instead of shaking hands, everyone could say hello to each other in different languages. Or everyone could do different high-fives to each other. High-fives, low-fives, round-the-back-fives. – make it different each time.

# Stuck in the mud

## ACTIVITY

This is a basic tag game. Choose someone to be It (or maybe more than one person, depending on the number of people playing). Everyone then runs around, away from It.

When a person is tagged, they must stand on the spot with their legs apart and arms out. They have to stay in that spot, in that position – stuck in the mud – until they are freed. A person is freed by another person running under their arms or through their legs. It's aim is to get everyone stuck in the mud.

## OTHER RULES

Change the number of Its. Limit the amount of space everyone can run around. Change how you move around. You don't always have to run – try skipping, jumping or hopping.

### EQUIPMENT
⭐ None

### WHERE
⭐ Anywhere with space to run around

### SAFETY TIPS
Remember to look where you're going. With younger kids, it is sometimes a good idea to get them all to move in the same direction to avoid collisions.

# Fruit corners

## ACTIVITY

Four cones are set out in a big square. Each cone represents a fruit: for example, a yellow cone could be a banana, a green cone could be an apple, a red one a strawberry and a blue one a blueberry. Someone is chosen to be the caller and they stand in the middle of the square. They cover their eyes and count to ten. Everyone runs to a cone. With their eyes still covered, the person in the middle calls out a fruit. Anyone at that cone is out. This continues until there is only one person left.

## OTHER RULES

Instead of running, everyone has to hop or skip to their cone. Hopping and skipping can be much more tiring than running.

### EQUIPMENT
⭐ 4 different-coloured cones or small objects

### WHERE
⭐ Outside

### SAFETY TIPS
If you are hopping or jumping between cones, remember to bend your knees each time you land. Hold your arms out to your sides to help you to keep your balance and stop you falling over.

## Myths

**MYTH:** It's a myth that you need to stretch before exercise. It won't improve your performance or reduce injury. Instead, warm up by building up your pace gradually.

## Facts

"If you release your energy playing with your family, everyone will sleep better!"

# Wink murder

## ACTIVITY

This is a 'chill out' game to play at the end of a more active session. Everyone stands in a circle. One person is chosen to be the detective, and they go and cover their eyes away from the circle. One person is then quietly chosen as the 'murderer'. Make sure no one says that person's name out loud or points them out to the detective, but ensure that everyone except the detective knows who the murderer is.

Everyone then calls for the detective to come to the middle of the circle by shouting, 'Detective, Detective, we need your help!' When the murderer winks at you, you must play dead. The detective then has three chances to guess who the murderer is. While 'alive', everyone except the detective has to jump up and down on the spot until the detective correctly identifies the murderer.

## OTHER RULES

Younger kids can poke their tongue out if they have problems winking. Hop on one leg or do star jumps instead of jumping on the spot.

| EQUIPMENT |
| --- |
| ⭐ None |

| WHERE |
| --- |
| ⭐ Anywhere |

# Monkey football

## ACTIVITY

Everyone stands in a circle with their feet apart and touching their neighbours' feet. The space between their feet is their goal. One person starts, and rolls the ball along the floor within the circle. The aim is to try to score a goal through someone else's legs.

Use your hands to stop the ball going through your legs for a goal. Once the ball has been rolled to you, it's your turn to try to score a goal. The winner is the player who scores ten goals first.

## OTHER RULES

Make it more difficult for anyone who lets in a goal. For example, they could be made to use only one hand to save goals until they make a save. Then they can go back to using two hands. Or make everyone start with their back to the centre. Try adding forfeits for people who throw the ball instead of rolling it.

| EQUIPMENT |
| --- |
| ⭐ Volley ball or other soft ball, or rugby ball for extra difficulty |

| WHERE |
| --- |
| ⭐ Anywhere with space |

**SAFETY TIPS**
Make sure the ball is rolled rather than thrown about the circle. Be careful when you roll the ball because it can move about the circle quite quickly.

# "When you don't want to go outside, balloon games are just the ticket for indoor activity!"

## PARTY GAMES

Have some balloon races. Get into two teams and form lines. Be the first team to move a balloon along the line using only your hands, or only your feet, head or chest. Try running with the balloon in your mouth, or between your feet, knees or ankles. Tie balloons to your ankles. Each team tries to burst the other's balloons. The team with the last whole balloon wins.

# Balloon-tastic!

Balloons are cheap, safe and great fun – and they always **remind you of parties**. They won't break your best china so they can be used **instead of balls** for indoor games on a **rainy day**.

**B**alloon games can be played on your own, in pairs, with friends or used for party games. Blow up a few balloons and start having fun. Invent your own games or use these three ideas for inspiration. The only limit is your imagination!

### BALLOON 8s

Time to be a basketball star! Stand with your legs apart and try to work a balloon around and through your legs in a figure-of-8 shape as fast as you can. Time yourself and see how many figure-of-8s you can do in one minute.

### BALLOONING AROUND

Hold a balloon between your legs and hop around with it. See how high you can jump with it between your legs. Or have a standing long-jump challenge and see how far you can jump from a standstill.

### BALLOON KEEPY-UPPY

Try to keep a balloon up in the air for as long as possible, like people do with a football. Use your hands first of all, then your feet and then your head. Finally, as the balloon floats downwards, try to balance it on your chest. Then you could start again!

# Home challenge for everyone

**I love a challenge** and there's nothing more motivating than trying to **achieve a goal**. Whether it's jumps, or skips or ball catches, it's good to set yourself a **personal target**. Better still, try to **beat someone else** in your family!

### PHYSICAL ACTIVITY AT HOME

Get your family to take part in activity challenges at home. Keep it simple – it's surprising how much fun you'll have once there's a bit of healthy competition!

- Can you get two, three or four others at home to do 100 skips each day for a week?
- Can you get two or more people at home to do 100 ball throws and catches each day for a week?
- Can you get two or more people at home to record their personal bests for a standing long-jump?
- Can you get everyone to spend 20 minutes dancing to their favourite music three times a week for six weeks?

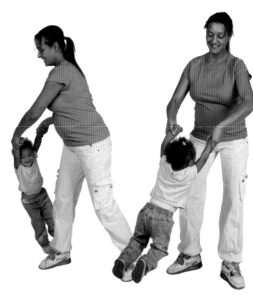

## SPEED CHALLENGES

Kids love challenges against the clock. Use a timer or a watch with a second hand and see who can run a certain distance and back in the quickest time. Or time kids doing 20 skips with a skipping rope or completing ten press-ups.

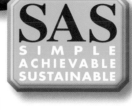

**SAS**
SIMPLE
ACHIEVABLE
SUSTAINABLE

### Bounce and catch
*Bounce a ball against a wall and catch it ten times? Now stand further away from the wall. That's harder!*

### Swing, hop or jump
*You don't need special equipment to keep fit. Assign a different fun activity to each room of your home. For example, five swings in the lounge, ten hops in the hall or five jumping jacks in the bedroom. Do these whenever you go in that room.*

# Keeping active

People are spending more and more time **sitting at a desk** in front of a computer screen. Everyone needs to make sure they **build activity** into every day – even while at the office – if they are to **stay healthy**.

**S**itting at a desk all day is not good for your health or your stress levels. Your body is not designed to hold this position for long periods of time. But it can be difficult to get away from the office to visit the gym or even to go for a walk.

### EXERCISE AT YOUR DESK

You can keep in shape by doing exercises at your desk. Try some of these during your next break between tasks:

- Let your head loll over so your right ear nearly touches your right shoulder. Using your hand, gently press your head a little lower. Hold for ten seconds. Relax, and repeat on the other side.
- Sitting tall in your chair, stretch both arms over your head and reach up. Hold for ten seconds then relax.
- Sitting in a chair, extend one leg out straight. Hold for two seconds then lower your foot and relax. Repeat ten times with each leg.

**1**

**2**

**Calf stretch**
*(1) From a standing position, take an exaggerated step forwards, keeping your back leg straight. Hold on to your desk and keep your arms straight but loose.*

*Your front knee should be at a 90° angle and above your foot. (2) Lean forwards so that your back leg and body make a continuous line. Count to ten then repeat with the other leg.*

**Tricep dips**
*Place your hands shoulder-width apart, fingers facing forwards, on the edge of a desk. Bend your elbows and lower your body until your elbows form a 90° angle. Hold for two seconds, then straighten your arms to bring you back up to the starting position. Aim for ten dips.*

# at work too!

## WORK STATION TOP TIPS

Try to do three or four exercises during every hour of continuous work – or as much as is possible and realistic. Try to stretch more frequently. Perform each stretch smoothly and SLOWLY, avoiding jerky movements. Keep a good posture, with relaxed shoulders and arms.

**SAS**
SIMPLE
ACHIEVABLE
SUSTAINABLE

## Thigh stretches

*Hold on to your desk for support. Stand straight, bend one leg behind you and hold the ankle. Count to ten, and then repeat on the other side.*

## Desk squats

*This is a simple exercise you can use to exercise your legs at work. Just face your desk and stand up. Then place your palms on the desktop and squat down until your thighs are parallel to the floor. Keep your back straight. Stand up again and repeat ten times.*

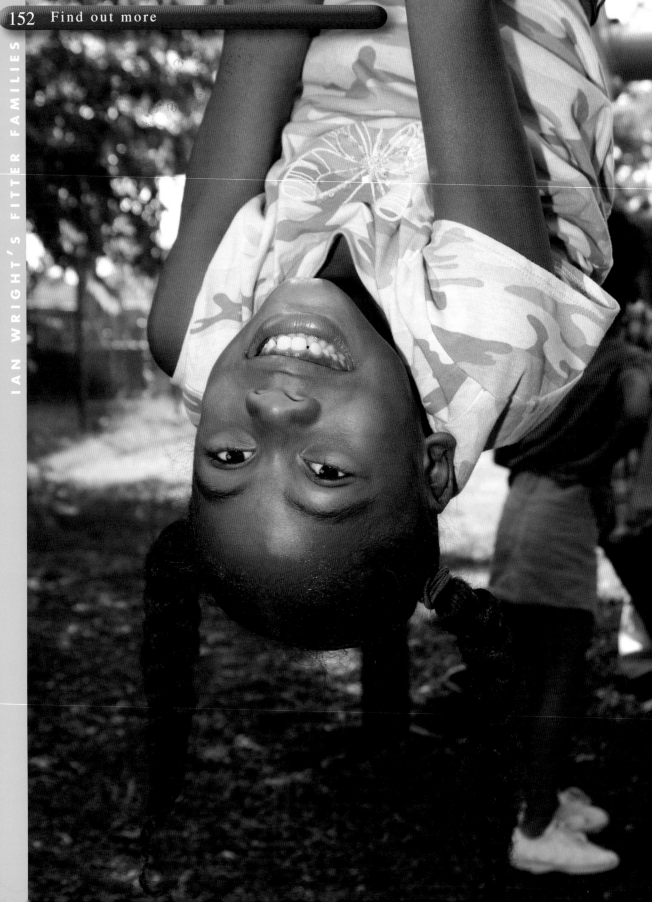

# Find out more

I hope that reading this book has **inspired** you to lead a **healthier lifestyle**, and encouraged you to become fitter by making activity part of your **daily routine**. Perhaps you've decided to take up a **new sport**, **join a club** or just **get out and walk more**. Whatever takes your fancy, there's plenty more information out there to help you **stay on track**.

*Myths & Facts*

**MYTH:** It's a myth that if your muscles aren't sore the next day, you didn't work out hard enough. Being sore for days after exercise means you overdid it.

# Useful websites

The aim of this section is to **point you in the right direction** if you want to know more about **sport, health, fitness or healthy eating**. Log on to one of the following websites – they are packed with **useful ideas and tips**.

### Fit For Sport
**www.fitforsport.co.uk** To help with your family's commitment to a healthy lifestyle, please visit our website and keep up to date with all the latest information so you can continue your SAS approach. Here you will also be able to purchase the Fitter Families Kit Bag, which will give you hours of family fun. Fit for Sport are the UK's leading children's healthy lifestyle activities provider. We are committed to delivering our promise of 'keeping the future fit' while educating our children and their families to live a healthy lifestyle.

### Great Run
**www.greatrun.org** Provides information for families on running events all year round. It has a section with training advice and how to plan your own training programme.

### Sport England
**www.sportengland.org** Has lots of inspiration and ideas on how to do more activity. Also has a database of over 15,000 locations in which to play sport, get fit and have fun!

### Sports Council for Wales
**www.sports-council-wales.co.uk** Official home of Welsh sport. Has lots of information on why and how to get involved in sport in Wales.

### Sport Scotland
**www.sportscotland.org.uk** Home of the national agency for sport in Scotland. Has a 'Get Active' section where you can find different sports facilities, plus a link to a database of sporting events across Scotland.

### Sports Council Northern Ireland
**www.sportni.net** Has information on sports organisations throughout Northern Ireland.

# "Find out what sporting activities are on near you – and get involved!"

IAN WRIGHT'S FITTER FAMILIES

**Food Standards Agency**
**www.eatwell.gov.uk** Has information to help you choose the right foods. Has an area specifically for children and teens.

**British Heart Foundation (BHF)**
**www.bhf.org.uk** Has information on how to stay fit, eat the right food and find events and activities. There is a specific section on kids' health.

**Everyday Sport**
**www.everydaysport.com** Provides details of sports activities that are going on near you. Also has a hotline (0800 587 6000).

**The Fit Map**
**www.thefitmap.com** Has articles about healthy living, interactive tools and details of health clubs and gyms throughout the UK.

**Food Fitness**
**www.foodfitness.org.uk** Offers practical advice on heathy eating and an active lifestyle. Contains 'It's your choice', a section for teenagers.

**British Nutrition Foundation**
**www.nutrition.org.uk** Has lots of useful information on nutrition tailored to people of all ages and levels of fitness.

**Active places**
**www.activeplaces.com** Lists thousands of places to play sport and get fit, from swimming pools and golf clubs to ice rinks and ski slopes.

**BBC Healthy living**
**www.bbc.co.uk/health/healthy_living** Provides good, clear information on lots of health, fitness and nutrition topics.

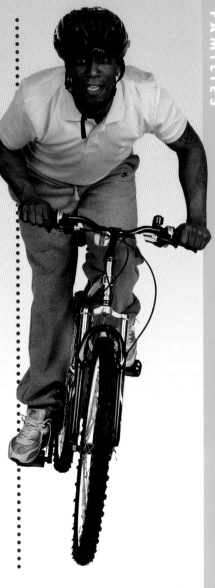

## BUPA – Physical Activity
**www.bupa.co.uk/health_information/asp/healthy_living/lifestyle/exercise** Packed with advice and details of how to be more active. Has lots of information on nutrition and health.

## Runner's World magazine
**www.runnersworld.co.uk** Has excellent articles on nutrition, training, sports injuries and sports nutrition product reviews.

## I want 2 be healthy
**www.iwant2behealthy.com** Discusses the importance of a good balanced diet for health and wellbeing. Looks at topics such as healthy eating, nutrition, obesity, cancer and heart disease.

## Join the Activaters
**www.jointheactivaters.org.uk** Fun website with games and information for parents, teachers and kids on how to get active and eat healthy food.

## Health Education Trust
**www.healthedtrust.com** An excellent resource for news and information on health for young people, with sections on school food and drink.

## BHF National Centre for Physical Activity and Health
**www.bhfactive.org.uk** Has advice, research and resources for professionals about physical activity and health at different stages in life.

## NHS Direct
**www.nhsdirect.nhs.uk** Gives information on healthy eating. You can also contact NHS Direct on 0845 4647.

## Walking the Way to Health
**www.whi.org.uk** Has everything you need to know about walking in England. Includes walking routes, training information and special events.

## Keep Fit Association
**www.keepfit.org.uk** Teaches safe and effective movement, exercise and dance classes for people of all ages and abilities.

## Wired for Health
**www.wiredforhealth.gov.uk** A series of websites managed on behalf of the Department of Health and the Department for Education and Skills. Provides health information that relates to the National Curriculum and the Healthy School Programme and supports a Whole School Food Policy.

**TOP TIPS**
It can be hard to keep going. Think about why you're trying to eat more healthily and be more active. Look back at your goals and remind yourself what you're trying to achieve for the whole family. Get fresh inspiration from these websites. And never give in – you can do better tomorrow!

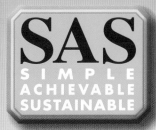

## Kids Health (The Nemours Foundation)
**www.kidshealth.org** US-based website that offers expert health nutrition and fitness advice for parents, kids and teenagers.

## British Dietetic Association
**www.bda.uk.com** Includes fact sheets and information on healthy eating for children. Also provides details of registered private dieticians.

## Healthy Living
**www.healthyliving.gov.uk/physicalactivity** Explains the benefits of physcial activity as part of a healthy lifestyle and gives advice on how to achieve the recommended level of exercise.

## DEFRA Country walks
**http://countrywalks.defra.gov.uk** Has details and maps for more than 1,800 walks, rides and areas of open access.

## The Ramblers Association
**www.ramblers.org.uk** Tells you about walking and helps you find local routes, walking events and walking groups.

## 5 a day
**www.5aday.nhs.uk** Has information about '5 a day' and what counts as a portion, as well as some top tips and a fun-and-games section.

## Men's Fitness magazine
**www.mensfitnessmagazine.co.uk** Contains lots of health and fitness tips and features. Has a print-friendly fitness test you can take and a workout archive to browse through.

## Prevention magazine
**www.prevention.com** US health and fitness magazine that promotes healthy living. Has lots of great tools and quizzes, latest news and research findings and online exercise programmes to follow.

## Weight Concern
**www.weightconcern.com** Has excellent information on obesity issues, including a section on children's health and a BMI (body mass index) calculator.

## National Register of Personal Trainers
**www.nrpt.co.uk** Has a fully searchable online database of qualified, insured and experienced UK personal trainers. Also has a forum.

# A final word

Now you've got all the information you need to become a **fitter family**. So, before you go and put your trainers on, here's a quick summary of my **main messages**.

⭐ Getting fit is all about making Simple, Achievable and Sustainable changes to your daily life. Decide which activities you will do and **stick to them**.

⭐ Set realistic goals and follow the **SMART** principles (see page 18).

⭐ Make a **commitment** to fitness. Put your goal in writing and you're more likely to achieve it.

⭐ Add activity to your daily life. **Start walking more**, taking the stairs, getting off the bus one stop earlier …

⭐ Do **whatever you enjoy** – gardening, walking, cycling to work, playing football with the kids. Just get moving!

⭐ Start gently and build up gradually. The changes will become a habit over time and **you'll hardly notice them**.

⭐ Think **fit for life**. Don't pressure yourself trying to achieve unrealistic goals. Take small steps to make your life as healthy as possible in a sustainable way.

⭐ Get the whole family involved and set a good example for your kids. When everyone joins in, it's easier to **keep going**.

⭐ Try to move your body at every opportunity. It **doesn't matter** for how long; the main thing is that you build a little more activity into your day.

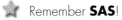 It is always good to vary the activities to **keep everyone interested** and their bodies challenged.

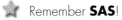 Don't diet. Let your children see that you enjoy healthy food and regular exercise. **Share mealtimes** as often as possible and eat the same foods.

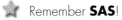 You can still eat your **favourite foods**, just a bit less of some of them – and more of others!

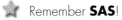 Remember **SAS**!

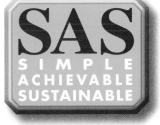

SAS
SIMPLE
ACHIEVABLE
SUSTAINABLE

# Acknowledgements

To all those people who worked so hard to make this book possible: a huge thank you. In particular, thanks go to Anita Bean and to the models: Laurence Payne, Michelle Horridge, Amy-May Payne, Lilly Payne, Terry Russell, Simone Waithe, Paris Waithe, Tyrelle Waithe, Armani Waithe Russell, and Baily Waithe Russell. Ian would also like to thank Stacey, Bobbie and his children who have been the inspiration for him to write this book. Dean would also like to thank his family – Karen, Dean, Charlie, Freya and William – for their support and efforts to be a fitter family, and Craig Jones at Fit For Sport for his inspirational ideas and energy.

The publishers would like to thank the following for their kind permission to reproduce their photographs:

b=bottom; c=centre; t=top; l=left; r=right

**7c** Guillermo Perales Gonzalez/iStockphoto; **8c** Tony Tremblay/iStockphoto; **9br** Heidi Kristensen/iStockphoto; **10bc** John Keith/iStockphoto; **11tc**, **11tl** Bookwork; **13c** Tony Tremblay/iStockphoto; **14c** Kelly Cline/iStockphoto; **14tl** iStockphoto; **15bc**, **19bc** Thomas Perkins/iStockphoto; **21c** Tony Tremblay/iStockphoto; **23cr** Olga Solovei/iStockphoto; **23tc** Graca Victoria/iStockphoto; **24c** Darren Baker/iStockphoto; **27bl** iStockphoto; **27tr** Lawrence Sawyer/iStockphoto; **28c** Marek Tarabura/iStockphoto; **30tl** Alexander Yakovlev/iStockphoto; **31c** Eileen Hart/iStockphoto; **32bc** Bonnie Jacobs/iStockphoto; **33tc** Leigh Schindler/iStockphoto; **35tc** En Tien Ou/iStockPhoto; **36c** Bonnie Jacobs/iStockphoto; **37bl** Kenneth C. Zirkel/iStockphoto; **37cr** Darren Baker/iStockphoto; **38cl**, **39cr** iStockphoto; **40c** Ilia Fuki/iStockphoto; **41br** Christine Balderas/iStockphoto; **42c** Arne Trautmann/iStockphoto; **44tr** Sergey Baykov/iStockphoto; **45c** Bonnie Jabobs/iStockphoto; **46cl** Chandra Widjaja/iStockphoto; **47bc** Pathathai Chungyam/iStockphoto; **50c** Bob Thomas/iStockphoto; **51c** Jaap Hart/iStockphoto; **52bl** Dieter Hawlan/iStockphoto; **52c** Jason Lugo/iStockphoto; **53c** Bonnie Jacobs/iStockphoto; **56c** Nikolay Suslov/iStockphoto; **57bl** iStockphoto; **60c** Dr Heinz Linke/iStockphoto; **62c** Ivan Batjic/iStockphoto; **64bl**, **64cl** Bookwork; **66c** Lisa Fletcher/iStockphoto; **66tr** iStockphoto; **67br** Christine Balderas/iStockphoto; **68cr** Bookwork; **69c** Nathan Gleave/iStockphoto; **70c** iStockphoto; **71br** David Hernandez/iStockphoto; **73c** Nikolay Suslov/iStockphoto; **73tr** Bookwork; **74bc** Angel Rodriguez/iStockphoto; **74cl** Bookwork; **74tc** Eric Gevaert/iStockphoto; **76tr** Bookwork; **77c** Juan Monino/iStockphoto; **78bl** Eric Delmar/iStockphoto; 78c Dane Steffes/iStockphoto; **79bc** Andrei Nekrassov/iStockphoto; **79tr** Eric Delmar/iStockphoto; **80c** Bookwork; **80cl** Kelly Cline/iStockphoto; **80tc** Nikolay Suslov/iStockphoto; **80tr** Bookwork; **81cr** Tomaz Levstek/iStockphoto; **82c** iStockphoto; **84br** Francesco Ridolfi/iStockphoto; **85cr** Nicole S Young/iStockphoto; **86tl** iStockphoto; **88c** Nicole S. Young/iStockphoto; **89br** Ivonne Wierink-vanWetten/iStockphoto; **90cr** Mark Jensen/iStockphoto; **90tr** Edyta Pawlowska/iStockphoto; **91tl** Alice Millikan/iStockphoto; **92tr** Andy Green/iStockphoto; **94cr** Elena Elisseeva/iStockphoto; **95c** Brad Killer/iStockphoto; **96c** iStockphoto; **98c** Nicole S. Young/iStockphoto; **99bc** iStockphoto; **100c** Martin Pernter/iStockphoto; **100cr**, **100tr** Bookwork; **102bl** Duncan Hotston/iStockphoto; **102tr** Helle Bro Clemmensen/iStockphoto; **103tc** iStockphoto; **104br**, **104cl**, **104cr**, **104tr** Bookwork; **105c** Ivan Mateev/iStockphoto; **106c** Miroslav Ferkuniak/iStockphoto; **110cl** Jaap Hart/iStockphoto; **112c** iStockphoto; **113br** Don Bayley/iStockphoto; **114bc** Rafa Irusta/iStockphoto; **114c** Sven Klaschik/iStockphoto; **116bl** Tony Robinson/iStockphoto; **117c** iStockphoto; **119c** Suprijono Suharjoto/iStockphoto; **120tc** Johannes Bayer/iStockphoto; **122bl** Eliza Snow/iStockphoto; **122tc** Bill Grove/iStockphoto; **124c** Miroslav Ferkuniak/iStockphoto; **127c** Tim Mccaig/ iStockphoto; **130c** Andrea Gingerich/iStockphoto; **134c** iStockphhoto; **144c** Heiko Potthoff/iStockphoto; **146c** Skip O'Donnell/iStockphoto; **148bl** Katrina Brown/iStockphoto; **152c** Bonnie Jacobs/iStockphoto; **156bc** Vladimir Melnikov/iStockphoto

All other photos © A&C Black